The
ECG Made Practical

The
ECG Made Practical

SEVENTH EDITION

JOHN HAMPTON DM MA DPhil FRCP FFPM FESC
Emeritus Professor of Cardiology, University of Nottingham, UK

DAVID ADLAM BA BM BCh DPhil FRCP FESC
Associate Professor of Acute and Interventional Cardiology and Honorary
Consultant Cardiologist, University of Leicester, Leicester, UK

ELSEVIER EDINBURGH LONDON NEW YORK OXFORD PHILADELPHIA ST LOUIS SYDNEY 2019

ELSEVIER

First edition 1986
Second edition 1992
Third edition 1997
Fourth edition 2003
Fifth edition 2008
Sixth edition 2013
Seventh edition 2019

The right of John Hampton and David Adlam to be identified as author(s) of this work has been asserted by them in accordance with the Copyright, Designs and Patents Act 1988.

Notices

Practitioners and researchers must always rely on their own experience and knowledge in evaluating and using any information, methods, compounds or experiments described herein. Because of rapid advances in the medical sciences, in particular, independent verification of diagnoses and drug dosages should be made. To the fullest extent of the law, no responsibility is assumed by Elsevier, authors, editors or contributors for any injury and/or damage to persons or property as a matter of products liability, negligence or otherwise, or from any use or operation of any methods, products, instructions, or ideas contained in the material herein.

ISBN 978-0-7020-7460-8
978-0-7020-7461-5

Printed in Scotland by Bell and Bain Ltd, Glasgow

Last digit is the print number: 9 8 7 6 5 4 3 2

Content Strategist: Laurence Hunter
Content Development Specialist: Fiona Conn
Project Manager: Louisa Talbott
Design: Brian Salisbury
Illustration Manager: Karen Giacomucci
Illustrator: Helius and Gecko Ltd

Contents

Preface   vii

12-lead ECGs   ix

1. The ECG in healthy people   1
2. The ECG in patients with palpitations and syncope: initial assessment   57
3. The ECG in patients with palpitations and syncope: ambulatory ECG monitoring   85
4. The ECG when the patient has a tachycardia   93
5. The ECG when the patient has a bradycardia   147
6. The ECG in patients with chest pain   195
7. The ECG in patients with breathlessness   255
8. The effects of other conditions on the ECG   283
9. Conclusions: four steps to making the most of the ECG   313

Index   317

Preface

What to expect of this book

This book is the seventh edition of *The ECG in Practice*, but we have changed the title to *The ECG Made Practical* to emphasize its relationship to *The ECG Made Easy*

We assume that the reader of this book will have the level of knowledge of the ECG that is contained in *The ECG Made Easy*. The ECG is indeed easy in principle, but the variations in pattern seen both in normal people and in patients with cardiac and other problems can make the ECG seem more complex than it really is. This book concentrates on these variations, and contains several examples of each abnormality. It is intended for anyone who understands the basics, but now wants to use the ECG to its maximum potential as a clinical tool.

The ECG is not an end in itself, but is an extension of the history and physical examination. Patients do not visit the doctor wanting an ECG, but come either for a health check or because they have symptoms. Therefore this book is organized according to clinical situations, and the chapters cover the ECG in healthy subjects and in patients with palpitations, syncope, chest pain, breathlessness or non-cardiac conditions. To emphasize that the ECG is part of the general assessment of a patient, each chapter begins with a brief section on history and examination.

This seventh edition continues the philosophy of its predecessors in that the patient is considered more important than the ECG. However, the ECG is a vital part of diagnosis and, increasingly, influences treatment. Electrical devices of various sorts are standard treatment in cardiology, and patients with such devices commonly present with non-cardiological problems. Those who are not specialists in cardiology need to

understand them so there is a series of changes in the text compared with previous editions: for example, there is more focus on ambulatory monitoring and newer monitoring devices and developments in pacing systems and defibrillators are described. We have made a clearer link between the ECGs of myocardial infarction, coronary anatomy and the site of myocardial injury. To make room for these changes, and to give more space to ECG interpretation, there is now less focus on patient management.

The new edition of the third title in the series is being published simultaneously and again we have changed the title, from *150 ECG Problems* to *150 ECG Cases* to emphasize the central place of the patient rather than the ECG. This new edition is divided into two sections, one containing numerous examples of 'everyday' ECGs which are suitable for those who have mastered *The ECG Made Easy*, and the other including more esoteric and difficult ECGs which provides more examples than can be included the this new edition of *The ECG Made Practical*. Those who want to practice their skills after reading *The ECG Made Practical* will find their challenge in the fifth edition of *150 ECG Cases*.

What to expect of the ECG

The ECG has its limitations. Remember that it provides a picture of the electrical activity of the heart, but gives only an indirect indication of the heart's structure and function. It is, however, invaluable for assessing patients whose symptoms may be due to electrical malfunction in the heart, especially patients with conduction problems and those with arrhythmias.

In healthy people, finding an apparently normal ECG may be reassuring. Unfortunately, the ECG can be totally normal in patients with severe coronary disease. Conversely, the range of normality is such that a healthy subject may quite wrongly be labelled as having heart disease on the basis of the ECG. Some ECG patterns that are undoubtedly abnormal (e.g. right bundle branch block) are seen in perfectly healthy people. It is a good working principle that it is the individual's clinical state that matters, not the ECG.

When a patient complains of palpitations or syncope, the diagnosis of a cardiac cause is only certain if an ECG is recorded at the time of symptoms – but even when the patient is symptom-free, the ECG may provide a clue for the prepared mind. In patients with chest pain the ECG may indicate the diagnosis, and treatment can be based upon it, but it is essential to remember that the ECG may remain normal for a few hours after the onset of a myocardial infarction. In breathless patients a totally normal ECG probably rules out heart failure, but it is not a good way of diagnosing lung disease or pulmonary embolism. Finally it must be remembered that the ECG can be quite abnormal in a patient with a variety of non-cardiac conditions, and one must not jump to the conclusion that an abnormal ECG indicates cardiac pathology.

Acknowledgements

In this seventh edition of *The ECG Made Practical* we have been helped by many people. In particular, we are grateful to our development editor, Fiona Conn, for her enormous attention to detail that led to many improvements in the text. We are also grateful to Laurence Hunter and his team at Elsevier for their encouragement and patience. As before, we are grateful to many friends and colleagues who have helped us to find the wide range of examples of normal and abnormal ECGs that form the backbone of the book.

JH, DA

12-lead ECGs

AAI pacing   Fig. 5.31
Accelerated idionodal rhythm   Fig. 1.47
Accelerated idioventricular rhythm   Fig. 1.28
Anorexia nervosa   Fig. 8.24
Aortic stenosis, severe, left ventricular hypertrophy
    with   Fig. 7.8
Aortic stenosis and left bundle branch block
    Fig. 7.6
Atrial fibrillation   Fig. 4.21, Fig. 4.22, Fig. 5.10
Atrial fibrillation, uncontrolled   Fig. 7.1
Atrial fibrillation and anterior ischaemia   Fig. 6.26
Atrial fibrillation and coupled ventricular
    extrasystoles   Fig. 7.2
Atrial fibrillation and inferior infarction   Fig. 4.37
Atrial fibrillation and left bundle branch block
    Fig. 4.26, Fig. 4.27
Atrial fibrillation and right bundle branch block
    Fig. 4.32
Atrial fibrillation and Wolff–Parkinson–White
    syndrome   Fig. 4.45
Atrial flutter and 1:1 conduction   Fig. 4.20
Atrial flutter and 2:1 block   Fig. 4.17
Atrial flutter and 4:1 block   Fig. 4.19
Atrial flutter and intermittent VVI pacing   Fig. 5.27
Atrial flutter and variable block   Fig. 5.9
Atrial flutter in hypothermia   Fig. 8.2
Atrial septal defect and right bundle branch
    block   Fig. 8.9

Atrial tachycardia   Fig. 4.16
Atrioventricular nodal re-entry tachycardia (AVNRT)
    and anterior ischaemia   Fig. 4.14, Fig. 6.27

Bifascicular block   Fig. 2.22
Biventricular pacing   Fig. 7.22
Broad complex tachycardia of uncertain origin
    Fig. 4.34, Fig. 4.35
Brugada syndrome   Fig. 2.14, Fig. 2.15

Chronic lung disease   Fig. 7.19
Complete heart block   Fig. 5.13
Complete heart block and Stokes–Adams attack
    Fig. 5.15
Congenital long QT syndrome   Fig. 2.12

DDD pacing, atrial tracking   Fig. 5.34
DDD pacing, atrial and ventricular pacing   Fig. 5.33
DDD pacing, intermittent   Fig. 5.35
Dextrocardia   Fig. 1.11
Dextrocardia, leads reversed   Fig. 1.12
Digoxin effect   Fig. 8.17
Digoxin effect and ischaemia   Fig. 6.41
Digoxin toxicity   Fig. 8.18

Ebstein's anomaly, right atrial hypertrophy and right
    bundle branch block   Fig. 8.8
Ectopic atrial rhythm   Fig. 1.8

Electrical alternans   Fig. 8.12
Exercise-induced ischaemia   Fig. 6.44
Exercise-induced ST segment depression   Fig. 6.46
Exercise testing, normal ECG Fig. 6.43, Fig. 6.45

Fallot's tetralogy, right ventricular hypertrophy
    in   Fig. 8.7
Fascicular tachycardia   Fig. 4.33
First degree block and left bundle branch block
    Fig. 2.20
First degree block and right bundle branch
    block   Fig. 2.21, Fig. 5.7, Fig. 5.14
Friedreich's ataxia   Fig. 8.26

His pacing   Fig. 5.31
Hyperkalaemia   Fig. 8.13
Hyperkalaemia, corrected   Fig. 8.14
Hypertrophic cardiomyopathy   Fig. 2.6, Fig. 7.11
Hypokalaemia   Fig. 8.16
Hypothermia   Fig. 8.3
Hypothermia, atrial flutter   Fig. 8.2
Hypothermia, re-warming after   Fig. 8.4

Intermittent VVl pacing   Fig. 5.26
Ischaemia, anterior   Fig. 6.24
Ischaemia, anterior and atrial fibrillation   Fig. 6.26
Ischaemia, anterior and AV nodal re-entry
    tachycardia   Fig. 6.27
Ischaemia, anterior and inferior infarction and right
    bundle branch block   Fig. 6.21
Ischaemia, anterior and possible old inferior
    infarction   Fig. 6.23
Ischaemia, anterior and right bundle branch
    block   Fig. 6.20
Ischaemia, anterolateral   Fig. 6.25

Ischaemia, digoxin effect and   Fig. 6.41
Ischaemia, exercise-induced   Fig. 6.44
Ischaemia, ?left ventricular hypertrophy
    Fig. 7.10
Ischaemia, probable   Fig. 7.9

Junctional tachycardia with right bundle branch
    block   Fig. 4.33

Left anterior hemiblock   Fig. 7.12
Left atrial hypertrophy   Fig. 2.7
Left atrial hypertrophy and left ventricular
    hypertrophy   Fig. 7.3
Left bundle branch block   Fig. 2.3, Fig. 6.17
Left bundle branch block and aortic stenosis
    Fig. 7.6
Left ventricular hypertrophy   Fig. 2.2, Fig. 6.34,
    Fig. 6.39, Fig. 7.5, Fig. 7.7, Fig. 8.6
Left ventricular hypertrophy and ?ischaemia
    Fig. 7.10
Left ventricular hypertrophy and left atrial
    hypertrophy   Fig. 7.3
Left ventricular hypertrophy and severe aortic
    stenosis   Fig. 7.8
Limb lead switch   Fig. 1.3
Lithium treatment   Fig. 8.22
Long QT syndrome, congenital   Fig. 2.12
Long QT syndrome, drug toxicity   Fig. 4.43

Malignant pericardial effusion   Fig. 8.11
Mediastinal shift   Fig. 1.22
Mitral stenosis and pulmonary hypertension
    Fig. 7.4
Myocardial infarction, acute anterior and old
    inferior   Fig. 6.16

Myocardial infarction, acute anterolateral, with left axis deviation   Fig. 6.8
Myocardial infarction, acute inferior   Fig. 6.2
Myocardial infarction, acute inferior and anterior ischaemia   Fig. 6.13
Myocardial infarction, acute inferior infarction (STEMI) and anterior NSTEMI   Fig. 6.15
Myocardial infarction, acute inferior and old anterior   Fig. 6.14
Myocardial infarction, acute inferior and right bundle branch block   Fig. 6.18
Myocardial infarction, acute lateral   Fig. 6.6
Myocardial infarction, anterior   Fig. 6.5
Myocardial infarction, anterior NSTEMI   Fig. 6.22
Myocardial infarction, anterolateral, ?age   Fig. 6.9
Myocardial infarction, evolving inferior   Fig. 6.3, Fig. 6.4
Myocardial infarction, inferior and atrial fibrillation   Fig. 4.37
Myocardial infarction, inferior and right bundle branch block   Fig. 6.18
Myocardial infarction, inferior and right bundle branch block and ?anterior ischaemia   Fig. 6.21
Myocardial infarction, inferior and right ventricular infarction   Fig. 6.12
Myocardial infarction, inferior and ventricular tachycardia   Fig. 4.38
Myocardial infarction, lateral (after 3 days)   Fig. 6.7
Myocardial infarction, old anterior   Fig. 6.10
Myocardial infarction, old anterolateral NSTE-ACS   Fig. 6.40
Myocardial infarction, old inferior (possible) and anterior ischaemia   Fig. 6.23
Myocardial infarction, old posterior   Fig. 6.35
Myocardial infarction, posterior   Fig. 6.11

Normal ECG   Fig. 1.10, Fig. 1.13, Fig. 6.43, Fig. 6.45
Normal ECG, accelerated idionodal rhythm   Fig. 1.47
Normal ECG, people of African origin   Fig. 1.41, Fig. 1.42
Normal ECG, child   Fig. 1.50
Normal ECG, ectopic atrial rhythm   Fig. 1.8
Normal ECG, exercise testing   Fig. 6.44, Fig. 6.46
Normal ECG, high take-off ST segment   Fig. 1.32
Normal ECG, junctional escape beat   Fig. 1.6
Normal ECG, left axis deviation   Fig. 1.49
Normal ECG, 'leftward' limit of normality   Fig. 1.17
Normal ECG, notched S wave (V_2)   Fig. 1.27
Normal ECG, P wave inversion   Fig. 1.8, Fig. 1.35
Normal ECG, P wave inversion (lead VR, VL)   Fig. 1.35
Normal ECG, partial right bundle branch block pattern   Fig. 1.34
Normal ECG, pre-exercise   Fig. 6.47
Normal ECG, R wave dominance (lead II)   Fig. 1.14
Normal ECG, R wave dominance (V_1)   Fig. 1.23, Fig. 7.17
Normal ECG, R wave dominance (V_3)   Fig. 1.21
Normal ECG, R wave dominance (V_4)   Fig. 1.19
Normal ECG, R wave dominance (V_5)   Fig. 1.20, Fig. 1.25
Normal ECG, R wave size   Fig. 1.14, Fig. 1.15
Normal ECG, right axis deviation   Fig. 1.16
Normal ECG, 'rightward' limit of normality   Fig. 1.15
Normal ECG, R–R interval variation   Fig. 1.4
Normal ECG, RSR^1 pattern   Fig. 1.26
Normal ECG, RSR^{1}S^1 pattern Fig. 1.27
Normal ECG, S wave dominance (V_3)   Fig. 1.19
Normal ECG, S wave dominance (V_4)   Fig. 1.20
Normal ECG, septal Q wave   Fig. 1.29, Fig. 1.49
Normal ECG, small Q wave   Fig. 1.30, Fig. 1.37

Normal ECG, ST segment, isoelectric and sloping
  upward   Fig. 1.31
Normal ECG, ST segment depression   Fig. 1.34
Normal ECG, ST segment depression
  (nonspecific)   Fig. 1.35
Normal ECG, ST segment elevation   Fig. 1.33
Normal ECG, T wave, peaked   Fig. 8.15
Normal ECG, T wave, tall peaked   Fig. 1.44
Normal ECG, T wave flattening   Fig. 1.43
Normal ECG, T wave inversion (lead III)   Fig. 1.37
Normal ECG, T wave inversion (lead V_1)   Fig. 1.37
Normal ECG, T wave inversion (lead V_2)   Fig. 1.40
Normal ECG, T wave inversion (lead V_3)   Fig. 1.41
Normal ECG, T wave inversion (lead VR)   Fig. 1.36
Normal ECG, T wave inversion (lead VR, V_1–V_2)
  Fig. 1.39
Normal ECG, T wave inversion in people of African
  origin   Fig. 1.41, Fig. 1.42
Normal ECG, U wave, prominent/large   Fig. 1.45,
  Fig. 1.46, Fig. 1.48

Pericardial effusion, malignant   Fig. 8.11
Pericarditis   Fig. 6.33
Pre-exercise normal ECG   Fig. 6.47
Prolonged QT interval due to amiodarone   Fig.
  2.13, Fig. 8.20
Pulmonary embolus   Fig. 6.29, Fig. 6.30, Fig. 6.31,
  Fig. 6.32, Fig. 7.20
Pulmonary hypertension and mitral stenosis   Fig. 7.4
Pulmonary stenosis   Fig. 8.5

Re-warming after hypothermia   Fig. 8.4
Right atrial hypertrophy   Fig. 7.14
Right atrial hypertrophy and right bundle branch
  block, in Ebstein's anomaly   Fig. 8.8

Right atrial hypertrophy and right ventricular
  hypertrophy   Fig. 7.15
Right bundle branch block and acute inferior
  infarction   Fig. 6.18
Right bundle branch block and anterior
  infarction   Fig. 6.19
Right bundle branch block and anterior
  ischaemia   Fig. 6.20
Right bundle branch block and atrial septal
  defect   Fig. 8.9
Right bundle branch block and inferior infarction,
  ?anterior ischaemia   Fig. 6.21
Right bundle branch block and right atrial
  hypertrophy, in Ebstein's anomaly   Fig. 8.8
Right ventricular hypertrophy   Fig. 2.4, Fig. 7.18
Right ventricular hypertrophy, marked   Fig. 7.16
Right ventricular hypertrophy in Fallot's
  tetralogy   Fig. 8.7
Right ventricular hypertrophy and right atrial
  hypertrophy   Fig. 7.15
Right ventricular outflow tract ventricular tachycardia
  (RVOT-VT)   Fig. 4.3, Fig. 4.41
RSR^1 pattern   Fig. 1.26, Fig. 2.14
RSR^1S^1 pattern   Fig. 1.27

Second degree block (2:1)   Fig. 5.12
Sick sinus syndrome   Fig. 5.2
Sinus arrhythmia   Fig. 1.4
Sinus bradycardia   Fig. 1.6, Fig. 5.1, Fig. 5.2
Sinus rhythm, after cardioversion   Fig. 4.18,
  Fig. 4.36
Sinus rhythm, in Wolff–Parkinson–White syndrome
  type A   Fig. 4.12
Sinus rhythm and left bundle branch block   Fig.
  4.25

Sinus rhythm and normal conduction, post-cardioversion   Fig. 4.36
Sinus tachycardia   Fig. 1.5
ST segment, nonspecific changes   Fig. 6.1
ST segment depression, exercise-induced   Fig. 6.46
Subarachnoid haemorrhage   Fig. 8.25
Supraventricular extrasystole   Fig. 1.7, Fig. 4.7
Supraventricular tachycardia   Fig. 4.11

T wave, nonspecific changes   Fig. 6.1
T wave, nonspecific flattening   Fig. 6.42
T wave, unexplained abnormality   Fig. 6.38
Thyrotoxicosis   Fig. 8.10
Torsade de pointes   Fig. 2.11
Trauma   Fig. 8.23
Trifascicular block   Fig. 2.23

Ventricular extrasystole   Fig. 1.9, Fig. 4.8
Ventricular extrasystoles, coupled and atrial fibrillation   Fig. 7.2

Ventricular fibrillation   Fig. 4.50
Ventricular tachycardia   Fig. 4.29, Fig. 4.30, Fig. 4.31
Ventricular tachycardia, fusion and capture beats   Fig. 4.39
Ventricular tachycardia and inferior infarction   Fig. 4.38
Ventricular tachycardia torsade de pointes   Fig. 2.11
VVI pacing, bipolar   Fig. 5.24
VVI pacing, intermittent   Fig. 5.26
VVI pacing, unipolar   Fig. 5.25
VVI pacing in complete block   Fig. 5.28

Wolff–Parkinson–White syndrome and atrial fibrillation   Fig. 4.45
Wolff–Parkinson–White syndrome type A   Fig. 2.8, Fig. 2.9, Fig. 4.12, Fig. 4.44, Fig. 6.36, Fig. 7.13
Wolff–Parkinson–White syndrome type B   Fig. 2.10, Fig. 6.37

The ECG in healthy people

1

Types of ECG	**1**
The 'normal' ECG	**2**
The normal cardiac rhythm	2
The heart rate	2
Extrasystoles	5
The P wave	9
The PR interval	13
The QRS complex	15
The ST segment	35
The T wave	39
The QT interval	47
The ECG in athletes	49
The ECG in pregnancy	52
The ECG in children	52
What is a 'normal ECG'?	53
What to do	**55**
Further investigations	55
Treatment of asymptomatic ECG abnormalities	55

The ECG is frequently used as a screening tool whether from a truly asymptomatic, apparently 'healthy', subject (e.g. for an employment medical) or as part of the battery of initial investigations in patients presenting with new symptoms of uncertain significance or cause. ECG findings should always be interpreted in the clinical context in which it was taken. Over-interpretation of normal variations in the ECG may lead to misdiagnosis and risk initiation of unnecessary investigations and inappropriate management. Understanding variations in the ECG that we can expect to find in completely healthy people is therefore a key prerequisite to the accurate interpretation of ECGs that appear 'abnormal'.

TYPES OF ECG

ECG traces come in many guises including continuous single channel heart monitoring, 3-lead rhythm assessment, and even internal electrograms obtained from implanted devices or during cardiac procedures. The most 'complete' external ECG is the traditional 12-lead trace (Fig. 1.1). Accurate lead position (Fig. 1.2) is key as misplaced leads change the appearances of the trace and may lead to misinterpretation. For example, limb lead switches can resemble abnormalities of the cardiac axis (Fig. 1.3), whilst alterations of chest lead position, for example due to displacement in obese patients or by breast tissue, may resemble cardiac rotation with delayed anterior R-wave progression (see Fig. 1.20).

THE 'NORMAL' ECG

The normal cardiac rhythm

Sinus rhythm is the only normal sustained rhythm (see Fig. 1.1). In young people the R–R interval is reduced (i.e. the heart rate is increased) during inspiration, and this is called sinus arrhythmia (Fig. 1.4). When sinus arrhythmia is marked, it may mimic an atrial arrhythmia. However, in sinus arrhythmia each P–QRS–T complex is normal, and it is only the interval between them that changes.

Sinus arrhythmia becomes less marked with increasing age of the subject, and is lost in conditions such as diabetic autonomic neuropathy due to impairment of vagus nerve function.

The heart rate

There is no such thing as a normal heart rate, and the terms 'tachycardia' and 'bradycardia' should be used with care. There is no point at which a high heart rate in sinus rhythm has to be called 'sinus tachycardia' and there is no lower limit for 'sinus bradycardia'. Nevertheless, unexpectedly fast or slow rates do need an explanation.

Sinus tachycardia

The ECG in Fig. 1.5 was recorded from a young woman who complained of a fast heart rate. She had no other symptoms, but was anxious. There were no other abnormalities on examination, and her blood count and thyroid function tests were normal.

Fig. 1.1

Normal ECG

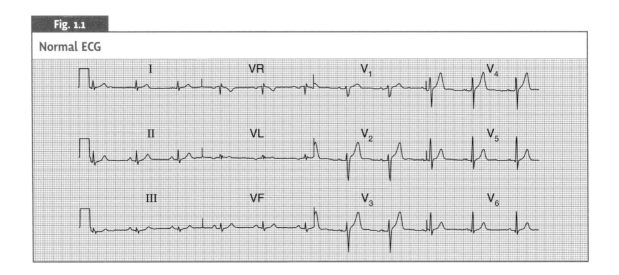

Fig. 1.2

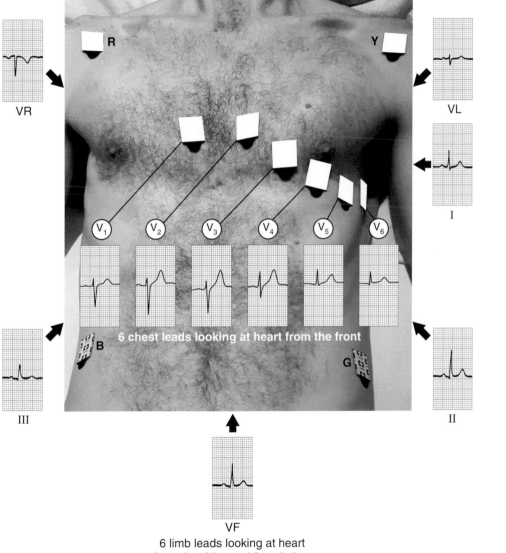

R

Y

VR

VL

I

V₁ V₂ V₃ V₄ V₅ V₆

6 chest leads looking at heart from the front

B

G

III

II

VF

6 limb leads looking at heart
from the sides and from below

ECG lead positions for the chest and upper limb leads. Correct positioning of the lower limb leads is also required for a 12-lead ECG (not shown here).

Fig. 1.3

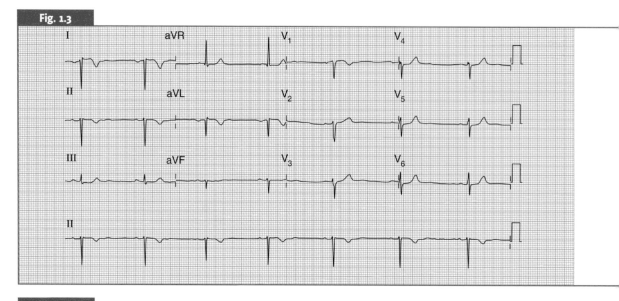

Fig. 1.4

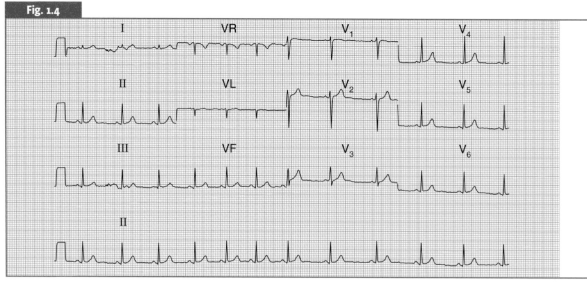

Limb lead switch

NOTE

- Prominent R wave in a VR
- Inverted limb lead complexes
- Normal chest leads

Sinus arrhythmia

NOTE

- Marked variation in R–R interval
- Constant PR interval
- Constant shape of P wave and QRS complex

BOX 1.1 Possible Causes of Sinus Rhythm With a Fast Heart Rate

- Pain, fright, exercise
- Hypovolaemia
- Myocardial infarction
- Heart failure
- Pulmonary embolism
- Obesity
- Lack of physical fitness
- Pregnancy
- Thyrotoxicosis
- Anaemia
- CO_2 retention
- Autonomic neuropathy
- Drugs:
  - sympathomimetics
  - salbutamol (including by inhalation)
  - caffeine
  - atropine

Box 1.1 shows possible causes of sinus rhythm with a fast heart rate.

Sinus bradycardia

The ECG in Fig. 1.6 was recorded from a young professional footballer. His heart rate was 44 bpm, and at one point the sinus rate became so slow that a junctional escape beat appeared.

The possible causes of sinus rhythm with a slow heart rate are summarized in Box 1.2.

Extrasystoles

Supraventricular extrasystoles, either atrial or junctional (atrioventricular [AV] nodal), occur commonly in normal people and are of no significance. Atrial extrasystoles (Fig. 1.7) have an abnormal P wave; in junctional extrasystoles either there is no P wave or the P wave may follow the QRS complex.

Fig. 1.5

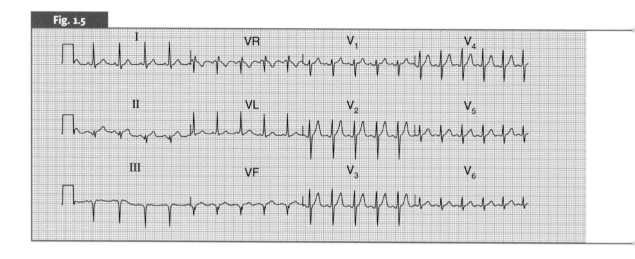

Fig. 1.6

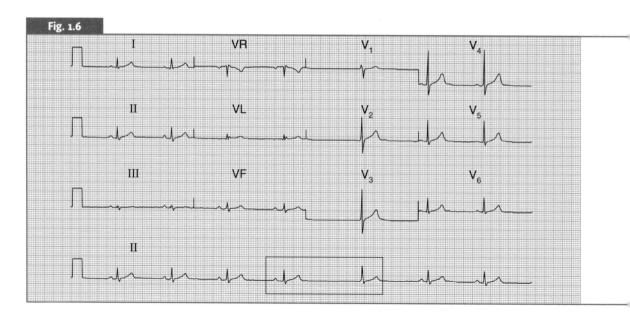

Sinus tachycardia

NOTE

- Normal P–QRS–T waves
- R–R interval 500 ms
- Heart rate 120 bpm

BOX 1.2 Possible Causes of Sinus Rhythm With a Slow Heart Rate

- Physical fitness
- Vasovagal attacks
- Sick sinus syndrome
- Acute myocardial infarction, especially inferior
- Hypothyroidism
- Hypothermia
- Obstructive jaundice
- Raised intracranial pressure
- Drugs:
  - beta-blockers (including eye drops for glaucoma)
  - calcium channel blockers (e.g. verapamil)
  - digoxin
  - ibabradine

In healthy people, normal sinus rhythm may be replaced by what are, in effect, repeated atrial extrasystoles. This is sometimes called an 'ectopic atrial rhythm' and it is of no particular significance (Fig. 1.8).

Ventricular extrasystoles are also commonly seen in normal ECGs (Fig. 1.9). Ventricular extrasystoles are almost universal, but when very frequent they indicate populations at increased risk and may merit further investigation (see Ch. 4, p. 101).

Sinus bradycardia

NOTE

- Sinus rhythm
- Rate 44 bpm
- One junctional escape beat

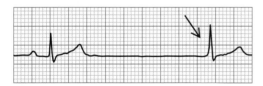

Junctional escape beat

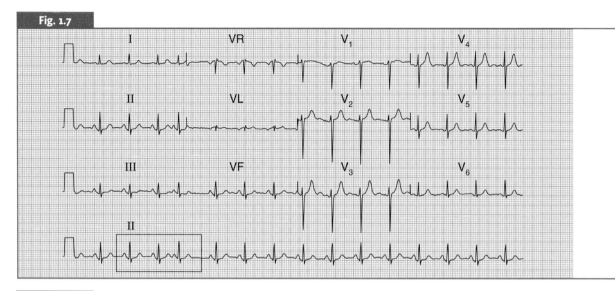

Fig. 1.7

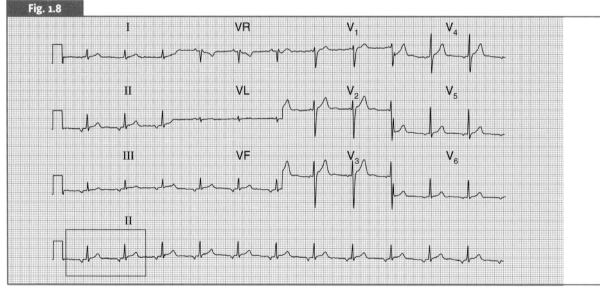

Fig. 1.8

Supraventricular extrasystole

NOTE

- In supraventricular extrasystoles the QRS complex and the T wave are the same as in the sinus beat
- The fourth beat has an abnormal P wave and therefore an atrial origin

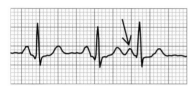

Early abnormal P wave

Normal variant: ectopic atrial rhythm

NOTE

- Sinus rhythm
- Inverted P wave in leads II–III, VF, V_4–V_6
- Constant PR interval

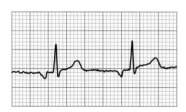

Inverted P waves in lead II

The P wave

In sinus rhythm, the P wave is normally upright in all leads except VR. When the QRS complex is predominantly downward in lead VL, the P wave may also be inverted (Fig. 1.10).

In patients with dextrocardia the P wave is inverted in lead I (Fig. 1.11). In practice this is more often seen if the limb leads have been wrongly attached (Fig. 1.3), but dextrocardia can be recognized if leads V_5 and V_6, which normally 'look at' the left ventricle, show a predominantly downward QRS complex.

Fig. 1.9

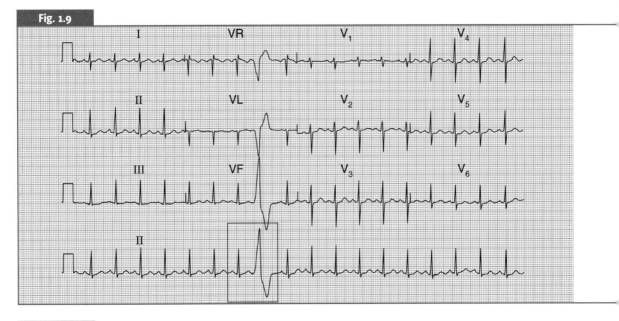

Fig. 1.10

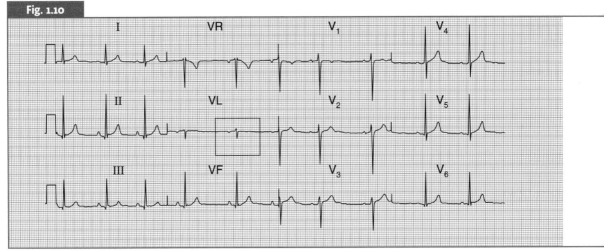

Ventricular extrasystole

NOTE

- Sinus rhythm, with one ventricular extrasystole
- Extrasystole has a wide and abnormal QRS complex and an abnormal T wave

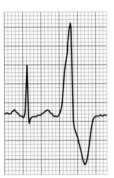

Ventricular extrasystole

Normal ECG

NOTE

- In both leads VR and VL the P wave is inverted, and the QRS complex is predominantly downward

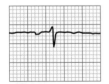

Inverted P wave in lead VL

If the ECG of a patient with dextrocardia is repeated with the limb leads reversed, and the chest leads are placed on the right side of the chest instead of the left, in corresponding positions, the ECG becomes like that of a normal patient (Fig. 1.12).

A notched or bifid P wave (P mitrale) is the hallmark of left atrial hypertrophy, and peaked P waves (P pulmonale) indicate right atrial hypertrophy – but bifid or peaked P waves can also be seen with normal hearts (Fig. 1.13) and are not particularly clinically useful features.

Fig. 1.11

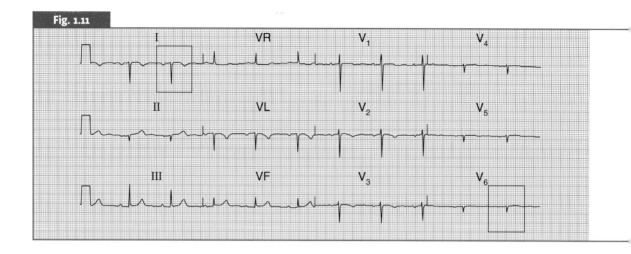

Fig. 1.12

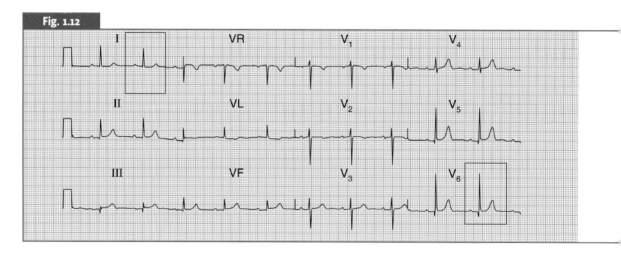

The PR interval

In sinus rhythm, the PR interval is constant and its normal range is 120–200 ms (3–5 small squares of ECG paper) (see Fig. 1.1). In atrial extrasystoles, or ectopic atrial rhythms, the PR interval may be short, and a PR interval of less than 120 ms suggests pre-excitation (see Figs 2.8, 2.9, 2.10).

A PR interval of longer than 220 ms may be due to first degree block, but the ECGs of healthy individuals, especially athletes, may have PR intervals of slightly longer than 220 ms – which can be ignored in the absence of any other indication of heart disease.

Dextrocardia

NOTE

- Inverted P wave in lead I
- No left ventricular complexes seen in leads V_5–V_6

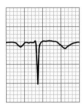 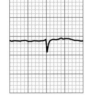

Inverted P wave and dominant S wave in lead I

Persistent S wave in lead V_6

Dextrocardia, leads reversed

NOTE

- Same patient as in Fig. 1.11
- P wave in lead I upright
- QRS complex upright in lead I
- Typical left ventricular complex in lead V_6

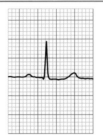 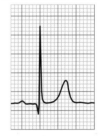

Upright P wave and QRS complex in lead I

Normal QRS complex in lead V_6

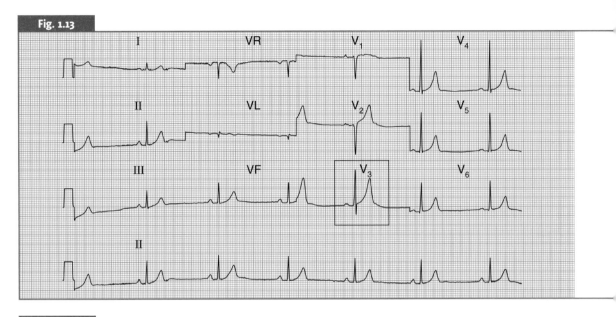

Fig. 1.13

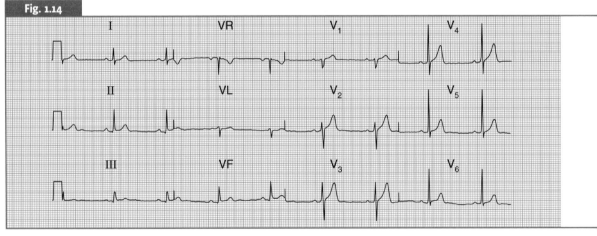

Fig. 1.14

Normal ECG

NOTE

- Sinus rhythm
- Bifid P waves, best seen in leads V_2–V_4
- Peaked T waves and U waves, best seen in leads V_2–V_3 – normal variants

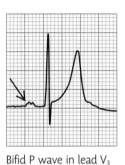

Bifid P wave in lead V_3

Normal ECG

NOTE

- QRS complex upright in leads I–III
- R wave tallest in lead II

The QRS complex
The cardiac axis

There is a fairly wide range of normality in the direction of the cardiac axis. In most people the QRS complex is tallest in lead II, but in leads I and III the QRS complex is also predominantly upright (i.e. the R wave is greater than the S wave) (Fig. 1.14).

Fig. 1.15

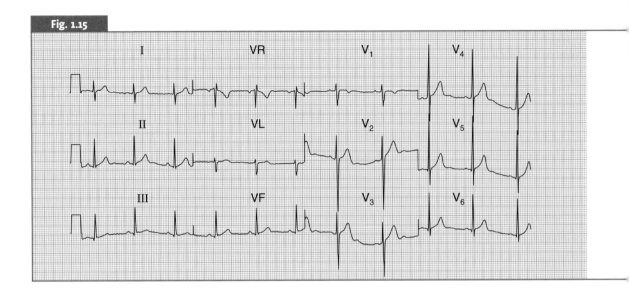

Fig. 1.16

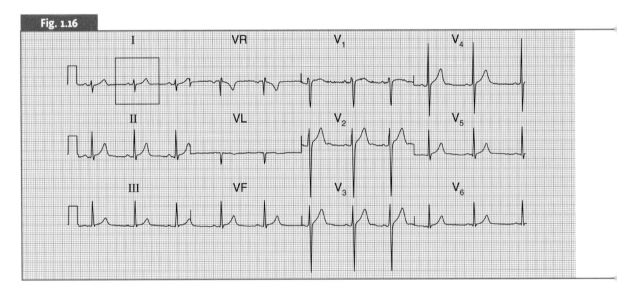

The cardiac axis is still perfectly normal when the R wave and S wave are equal in lead I: this is common in tall people (Fig. 1.15).

When the S wave is greater than the R wave in lead I, right axis deviation is present. However, this is very common in perfectly normal people. The ECG in Fig. 1.16 is from a professional footballer.

It is common for the S wave to be greater than the R wave in lead III, and the cardiac axis can still be considered normal when the S wave equals the R wave in lead II (Fig. 1.17). These patterns are common in obese people and during pregnancy.

When the depth of the S wave exceeds the height of the R wave in lead II, left axis deviation is present (see Figs 2.22 and 2.23).

Limb lead switches can sometimes be misinterpreted as abnormalities of cardiac axis (see Fig. 1.3).

Normal ECG

NOTE

- This record shows the 'rightward' limit of normality of the cardiac axis
- R and S waves equal in lead I

Normal ECG

NOTE

- Right axis deviation: S wave greater than R wave in lead I
- Upright QRS complexes in leads II–III

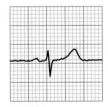

Dominant S wave
in lead I

Fig. 1.17

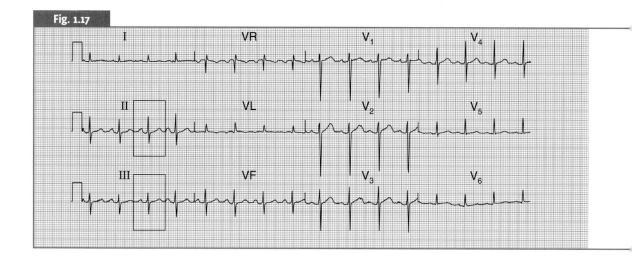

Fig. 1.18

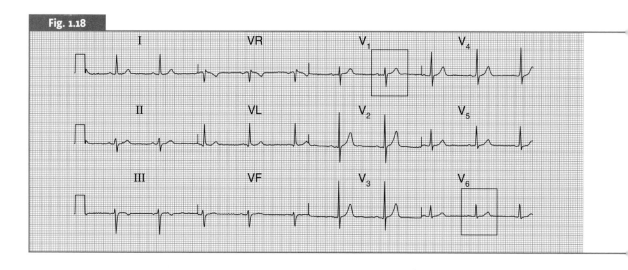

Normal ECG

NOTE

- This shows the 'leftward limit' of normality of the cardiac axis
- S wave equals R wave in lead II
- S wave greater than R wave in lead III

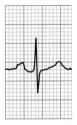
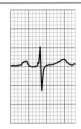

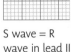

S wave = R
wave in lead II

S wave > R
wave in lead III

Normal ECG

NOTE

- Lead V_1 shows a predominantly downward complex, with the S wave greater than the R wave
- Lead V_6 shows an upright complex, with a dominant R wave and a tiny S wave

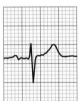
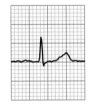

S wave > R wave in lead V_1 Dominant R wave in lead V_6

The size of R and S waves in the chest leads

In lead V_1 there should be a small R wave and a deep S wave, and the balance between the two should change progressively from V_1 to V_6. In lead V_6 there should be a tall R wave and no S wave (Fig. 1.18).

Typically the 'transition point', when the R and S waves are equal, is seen in lead V_3 or V_4 but there is quite a lot of variation. Fig. 1.19 shows an ECG in which the transition point is somewhere between leads V_3 and V_4.

Fig. 1.20 shows an ECG with a transition point between leads V_4 and V_5, and Fig. 1.21 shows an ECG with a transition point between leads V_2 and V_3.

The transition point is typically seen in lead V_5 or even V_6 in patients with chronic lung disease (see Ch. 7), and this is called 'clockwise rotation'. In extreme cases, the chest leads need to be placed in the posterior axillary line, or even further round to the back (leads V_7–V_9) before the transition point is demonstrated. A similar ECG pattern

Fig. 1.19

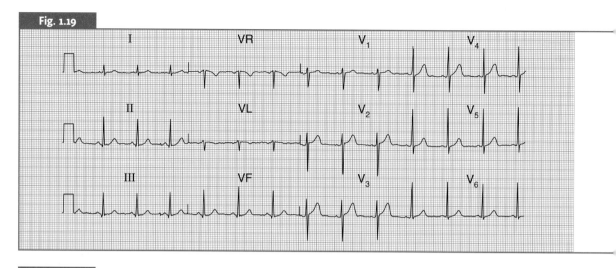

Fig. 1.20

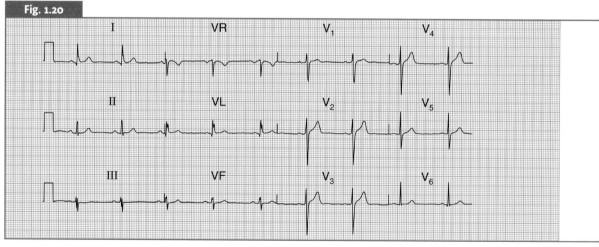

Normal ECG
NOTE

Normal ECG

NOTE

- In lead V_3 there is a dominant S wave
- In lead V_4 there is a dominant R wave
- The transition point is between leads V_3 and V_4

Normal ECG

NOTE

- Dominant S wave in lead V_4
- R wave just bigger than S wave in lead V_5

may be seen in patients with an abnormal chest shape, particularly when depression of the sternum shifts the mediastinum to the left. The patient from whom the ECG in Fig. 1.22 was recorded had mediastinal shift. An apparent 'clockwise rotation' ECG pattern can sometimes arise from lateral displacement of the ECG chest leads, particularly in larger patients or by breast tissue.

Occasionally the ECG of a totally normal subject will show a 'dominant' R wave (i.e. the height of the R wave exceeds the depth of the S wave) in lead V_1. There will thus, effectively, be no transition point, and this is called 'counterclockwise rotation'. The ECG in Fig. 1.23 was recorded from a healthy footballer with a normal heart. However, a dominant R wave in lead V_1 is usually due to either right ventricular hypertrophy (see Ch. 7) or a true posterior infarction (see Ch. 6).

Excessive R wave voltages may be an indication of left ventricular hypertrophy (see page 263). Provided that the ECG is properly calibrated (1 mV causes 1 cm of vertical deflection on the ECG), the limits for the sizes of the R and S waves in normal subjects are usually said to be:

- 25 mm for the R wave in lead V_5 or V_6
- 25 mm for the S wave in lead V_1 or V_2
- Sum of R wave in lead V_5 or V_6 plus S wave in lead V_1 or V_2 should be less than 35 mm.

However, R waves taller than 25 mm are commonly seen in leads V_5–V_6 in fit and thin young people, and are perfectly normal. Thus, once again, interpretation of these 'limits' depends on the clinical context. The ECGs in Figs 1.24 and 1.25 were both recorded from fit young men with normal hearts.

Fig. 1.21

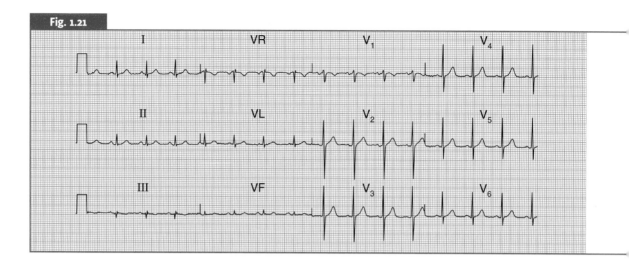

Fig. 1.22

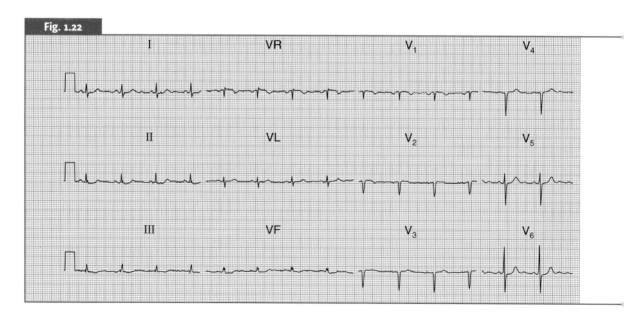

Normal ECG
NOTE
- Dominant S wave in lead V_2
- Dominant R wave in lead V_3
- The transition point is between leads V_2 and V_3

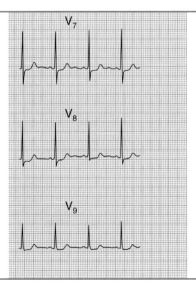

Mediastinal shift
NOTE
- 'Abnormal' ECG, but a normal heart
- Shift of the mediastinum means that the transition point is under lead V_6
- Ventricular complexes are shown in leads round the left side of the chest, in positions V_7–V_9

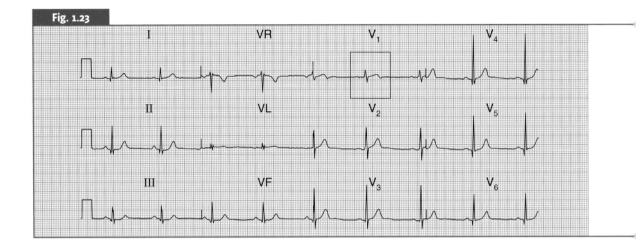

Fig. 1.23

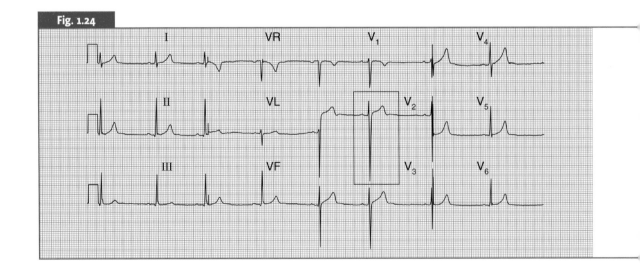

Fig. 1.24

Normal ECG
NOTE

- Dominant R waves in lead V_1

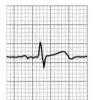

Dominant R wave
in lead V_1

Normal ECG
NOTE

- S wave in lead V_2 is 36 mm

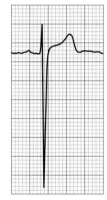

S wave > 25 mm in lead V_2

Fig. 1.25

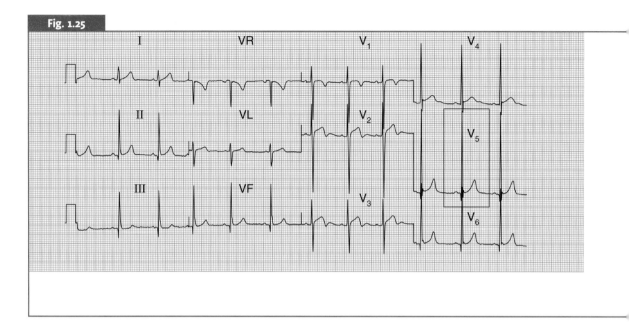

Fig. 1.26

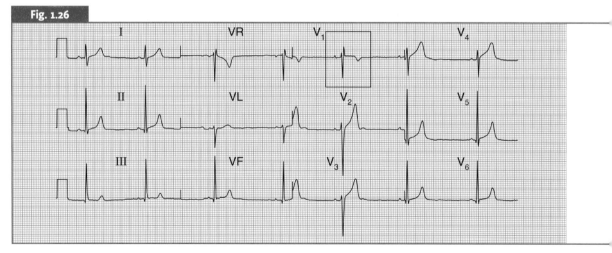

The width of the QRS complex

The QRS complex should be less than 120 ms in duration (i.e. less than 3 small squares) in all leads. If it is longer than this, then either the ventricles have been depolarized from a ventricular rather than a supraventricular focus (i.e. a ventricular rhythm is present), or there is an abnormality of conduction within the ventricles. The latter is most commonly due to bundle branch block. An RSR¹ pattern, resembling that of right bundle branch block (RBBB) but with a narrow QRS complex, is sometimes called 'partial right bundle branch block' and is a normal variant (Fig. 1.26). An RSRV pattern is also a normal variant (Fig. 1.27) and is sometimes called a 'splintered' complex.

In perfectly normal hearts the normal rhythm may be replaced by an accelerated idioventricular rhythm, which looks like a run of regular ventricular extrasystoles, with wide QRS complexes (Fig. 1.28).

Normal ECG
NOTE
- R wave in lead V_5 is 42 mm

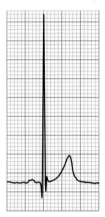

R wave > 25 mm in lead V_5

Normal ECG
NOTE
- RSR¹ pattern in lead V_2
- QRS complex duration 100 ms
- Partial right bundle branch block pattern

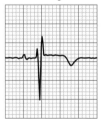

RSR¹ pattern and QRS complex 100 ms in lead V_1

Fig. 1.27

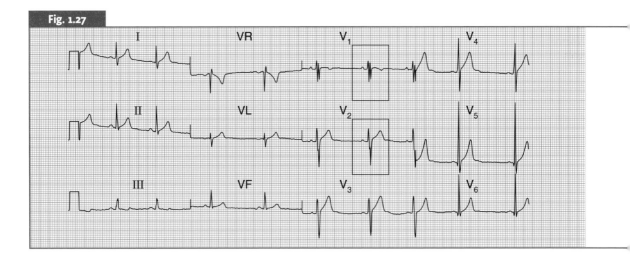

Fig. 1.28

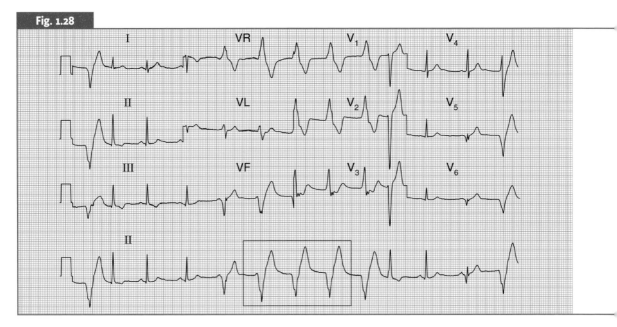

Normal ECG
NOTE
- RSR^{1}S^1 pattern in lead V$_1$
- Notched S wave in lead V$_2$
- QRS complex duration 100 ms
- Partial right bundle branch block pattern

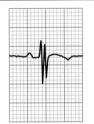 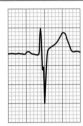

RSR^{1}S^1 pattern in lead V$_1$

Notched S wave in lead V$_2$

Accelerated idioventricular rhythm
NOTE
- Sinus rhythm
- First and last beats are ventricular extrasystoles
- The fifth beat starts a run of ventricular rhythm at about 80 bpm

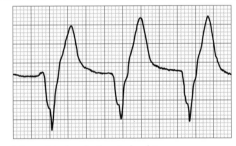

Idioventricular rhythm in lead II

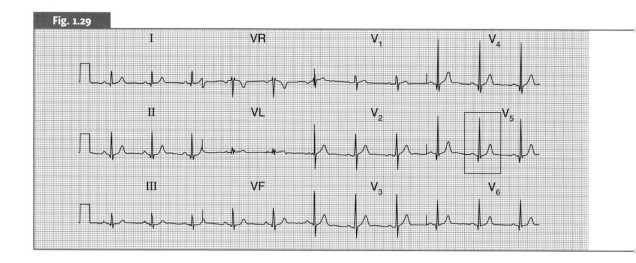

Fig. 1.29

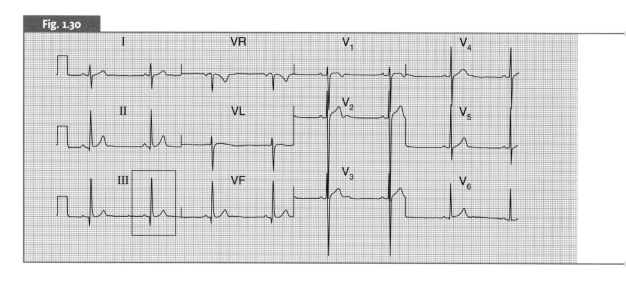

Fig. 1.30

Normal ECG

NOTE

- Septal Q waves in leads I, II, V_4–V_6

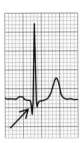

Septal Q wave in lead V_5

Normal ECG

NOTE

- Narrow but quite deep Q wave in lead III
- Smaller Q wave in lead VF

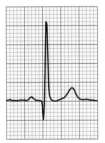

Narrow Q wave in lead III

Q waves

The normal depolarization of the interventricular septum from left to right causes a small 'septal' Q wave in any of leads II, VL, or V_5–V_6. Septal Q waves are usually less than 3 mm deep and less than 1 mm across (Fig. 1.29).

A small Q wave is also common in lead III in normal people, in which case it is always narrow but can be more than 3 mm deep. Occasionally, there will be a similar Q wave in lead VF (Fig. 1.30). These 'normal' Q waves become much less deep, and may disappear altogether, on deep inspiration (see Fig. 1.38.)

Fig. 1.31

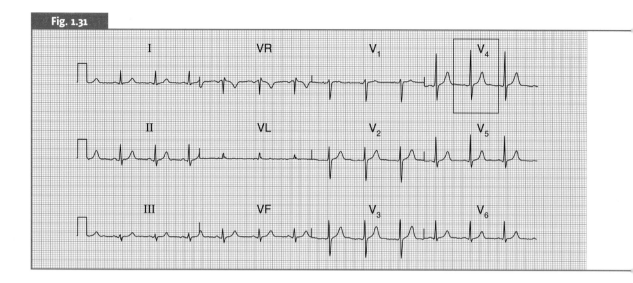

Fig. 1.32

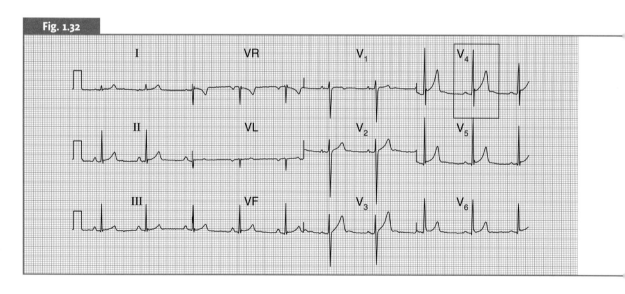

Normal ECG

NOTE

- ST segment is isoelectric but slopes upwards in leads V_2–V_5

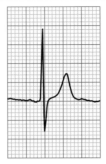

Upward-sloping ST segment in lead V_4

Normal ECG

NOTE

- In lead V_4 there is an S wave followed by a raised ST segment. This is a 'high take-off' ST segment

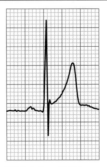

High take-off ST segment in lead V_4

Fig. 1.33

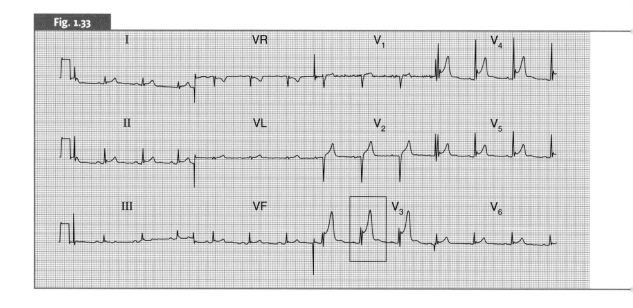

BOX 1.3 Causes of ST Segment Elevation Other Than Myocardial Infarction

- Normal variants (high take-off and early repolarization)
- Left bundle branch block
- Acute pericarditis and myocarditis
- Hyperkalaemia
- Brugada syndrome
- Arrhythmogenic right ventricular cardiomyopathy
- Pulmonary embolism

Normal ECG

NOTE

- Marked ST segment elevation in lead V_3 follows an S wave

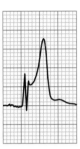

High take-off ST segment in lead V_3

The ST segment

The ST segment (the part of the ECG between the S wave and the T wave) should be horizontal and 'isoelectric', which means that it should be at the same level as the baseline of the record between the end of the T wave and the next P wave. However, in the chest leads the ST segment often slopes upwards and is not easy to define (Fig. 1.31).

An elevation of the ST segment is the hallmark of an acute myocardial infarction (see Ch. 6), and depression of the ST segment can indicate ischaemia or the effect of digoxin. However, it is perfectly normal for the ST segment to be elevated following an S wave in leads V_2–V_5. This is sometimes called a 'high take-off ST segment'. The ECGs in Figs 1.32 and 1.33 were recorded from perfectly healthy young men.

The ST segment is apparently raised when there is 'early repolarization', which causes the ST segment to be arched, and is usually only seen in the anterior leads, not the limb leads (see Fig. 1.41).

Box 1.3 shows the possible causes of ST segment elevation, other than myocardial infarction.

ST segment depression is measured relative to the baseline (between the T and P waves), 60–80 ms after the 'J' point, which is the point of inflection at the junction of the S wave and the ST segment. Minor depression of the ST segment is not uncommon in normal people, and is then called 'nonspecific'; the advantage of using this term is that it leaves the way open for a later change of diagnosis. ST segment depression in lead III but not VF is likely to be nonspecific (Fig. 1.34). Nonspecific ST segment depression should not be more than 2 mm (Fig. 1.35), and the segment often slopes upwards. Horizontal ST segment depression of more than 2 mm indicates ischaemia (see Ch. 6).

Fig. 1.34

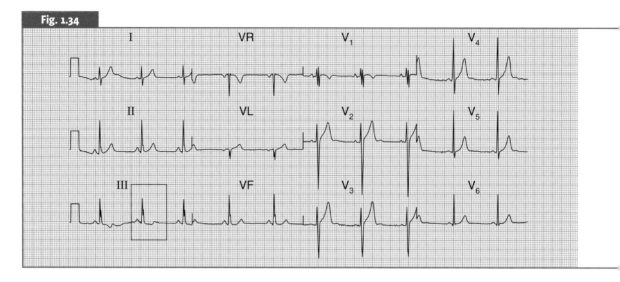

Fig. 1.35

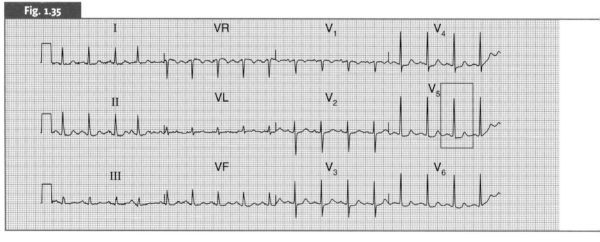

Normal ECG

NOTE

- ST segment depression in lead III but not VF
- Biphasic T wave (i.e. initially inverted but then upright) in lead III but not VF
- Partial right bundle branch block pattern

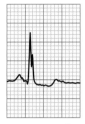

ST segment depression and biphasic T wave in lead III

Possibly normal ECG

NOTE

- ST segment depression of 1 mm in leads V_3–V_6
- In a patient with chest pain this would raise suspicions of ischaemia but, particularly in women, such changes can be nonspecific

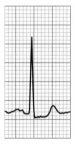

Nonspecific ST segment depression in lead V_5

Fig. 1.36

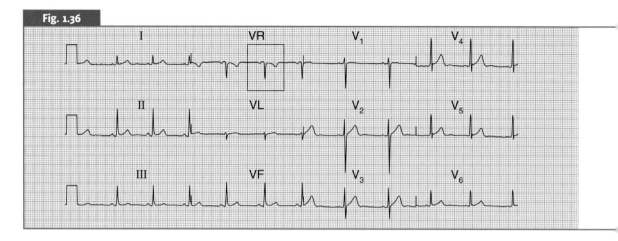

Fig. 1.37

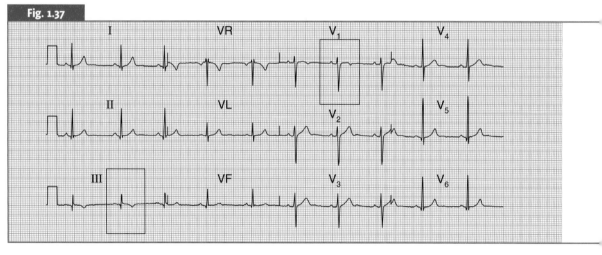

The T wave

In a normal ECG the T wave is always inverted in lead VR, and often in lead V_1, but is usually upright in all the other leads (Fig. 1.36).

The T wave is also often inverted in lead III but not VF. However, its inversion in lead III may be reversed on deep inspiration (Figs 1.37 and 1.38).

Normal ECG

NOTE

- T wave is inverted in lead VR but is upright in all other leads

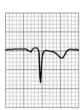

Inverted T wave in lead VR

Normal ECG

NOTE

- Small Q wave in lead III but not VF
- Inverted T wave in lead III but upright T wave in VF
- Inverted T wave in lead V_1

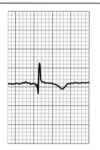

Q wave and inverted T wave in lead III

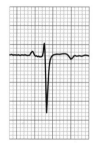

Inverted T wave in lead V_1

Fig. 1.38

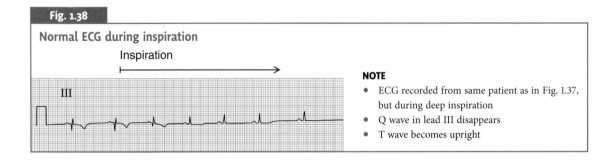

Normal ECG during inspiration

NOTE
- ECG recorded from same patient as in Fig. 1.37, but during deep inspiration
- Q wave in lead III disappears
- T wave becomes upright

Fig. 1.39

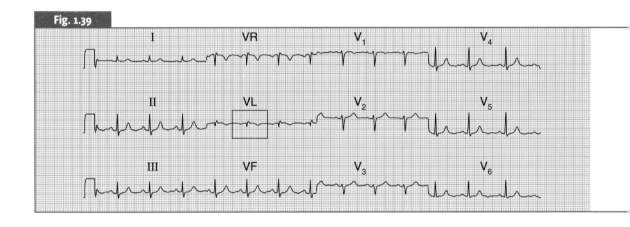

T-wave inversion in lead VL as well as in VR can be normal, particularly if the P wave in lead VL is inverted. The ECG in Fig. 1.39 was recorded from a completely healthy young woman.

T-wave inversion in leads V_2–V_3 as well as in V_1 occurs in pulmonary embolism and in right ventricular hypertrophy (see Chs 6 and 7), but it can be a normal variant. This is particularly true in people of African origin. The ECG in Fig. 1.40 was recorded from a healthy young Caucasian man, and that shown in Fig. 1.41 from a young black professional footballer. The ECG in Fig. 1.42 was recorded from a middle-aged woman of African origin with rather nonspecific chest pain, whose coronary arteries and left ventricle were shown to be entirely normal on catheterization.

Box 1.4 summarizes the situations in which T-wave inversion is seen.

Generalized flattening of the T waves with a normal QT interval is best described as 'nonspecific'. In a patient without symptoms and whose heart is clinically normal, the finding has little prognostic significance. This was the case with the patient whose ECG is shown in Fig. 1.43. In patients with symptoms suggestive of cardiovascular disease, however, such an ECG would require further investigation.

Normal ECG

NOTE

- Inverted T waves in leads VR, VL
- Inverted P waves in leads VR, VL

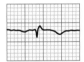

Inverted P and T waves in lead VL

BOX 1.4 Causes of T-Wave Inversion

- Normal in leads VR, V_1–V_2, and V_3, in people of African origin
- Normal in lead III when the T wave in lead VF is upright
- Ventricular extrasystoles and other ventricular rhythms
- Bundle branch block (right or left)
- Myocardial infarction
- Right or left ventricular hypertrophy
- Wolff–Parkinson–White syndrome

Fig. 1.40

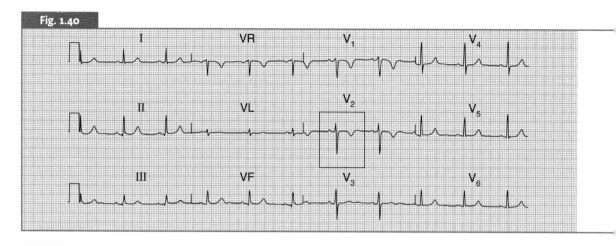

Fig. 1.41

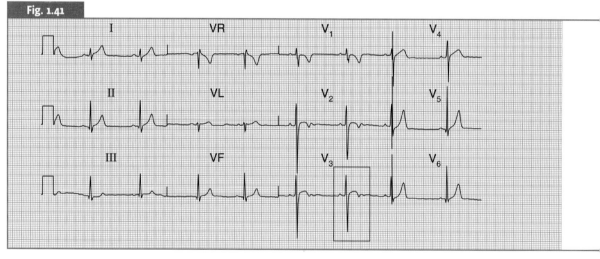

Normal ECG
NOTE

- T-wave inversion in leads VR, V_1–V_2
- Biphasic T wave in lead V_3

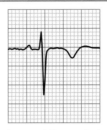

Inverted T wave in lead V_2

Normal ECG, from a man of African origin
NOTE

- T-wave inversion in leads VR, V_1–V_3
- Early repolarization in leads V_2–V_3

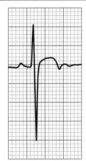

Inverted T wave in lead V_3

Fig. 1.42

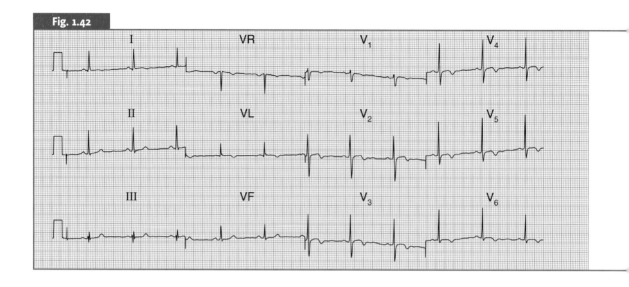

Fig. 1.43

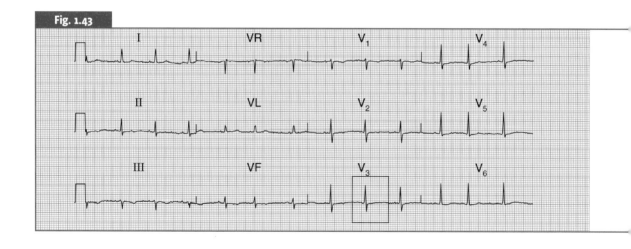

Normal ECG, from a woman of African origin
NOTE
- Sinus rhythm
- T-wave inversion in lead VL and all chest leads
- Presumably a normal variant: coronary angiography and echocardiography were normal

Possibly normal ECG
NOTE
- Sinus rhythm
- Normal axis
- Normal QRS complexes
- T-wave flattening in all chest leads
- T-wave inversion in leads III, VF
- In an asymptomatic patient, these changes are not necessarily significant

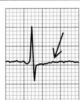

Flattened T wave in lead V₃

Fig. 1.44

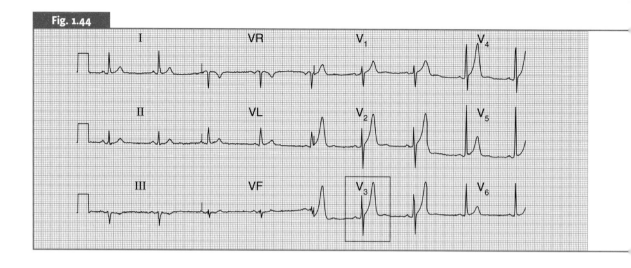

Fig. 1.45

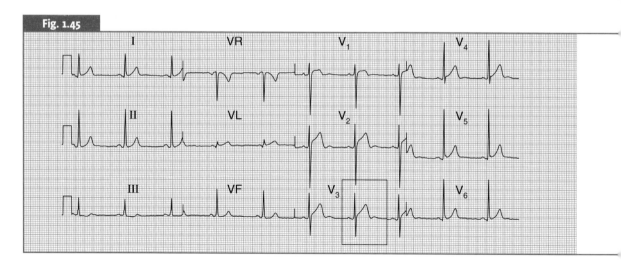

Peaked T waves are one of the features of hyperkalae-mia (see Fig. 8.13), but they can also be very prominent in healthy people (Fig. 1.44). Tall and peaked T waves are sometimes seen in the early stages of a myocardial infarction, when they are described as 'hyperacute'. They are, however, an extremely unreliable sign of infarction.

The T wave is the most variable part of the ECG. It may become inverted in some leads simply by hyperventilation associated with anxiety.

An extra hump on the end of the T wave, a 'U' wave, is characteristic of hypokalaemia. However, U waves are commonly seen in the anterior chest leads of normal ECGs (Fig. 1.45), where they can be remarkably prominent (Fig. 1.46). It is thought that they represent repolarization of the papillary muscles. A U wave is probably only important if it follows a flat T wave.

The QT interval

The QT interval (from the Q wave to the end of the T wave) varies with the heart rate, gender and time of day. There are several different ways of correcting the QT interval for heart rate, but the simplest is Bazett's formula. In this, the corrected QT interval (QT_C) is calculated as:

$$QT_C = \frac{QT}{\sqrt{(R-R \text{ interval})}}$$

An alternative is Fridericia's correction, in which QT_C is the QT interval divided by the cube root of the R–R interval. It is uncertain which of the corrections is clinically more important.

The upper limit of the normal QT_C interval is longer in women than in men, and increases with age. Its precise limit is uncertain, but is usually taken (following Bazett's correction) as 450 ms for adult men and 470 ms for adult women. Abnormal QT intervals may be associated with malignant arrhythmias and/or drug toxicity (see pages 72 and 302).

Normal ECG

NOTE

- Sinus rhythm
- Normal axis
- Normal QRS complexes
- Very tall and peaked T wave

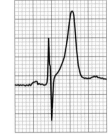

Tall peaked T wave in lead V_3

Normal ECG

NOTE

- Prominent U waves following normal T waves in leads V_2–V_4

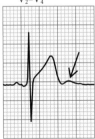

U wave in lead V_3

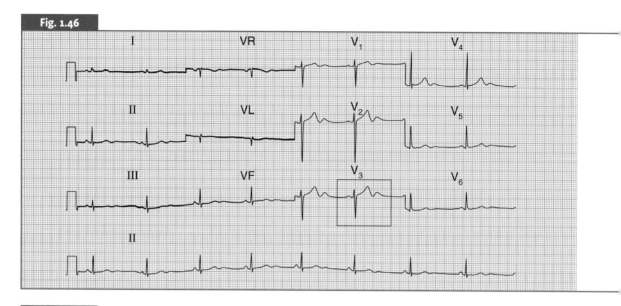

Fig. 1.46

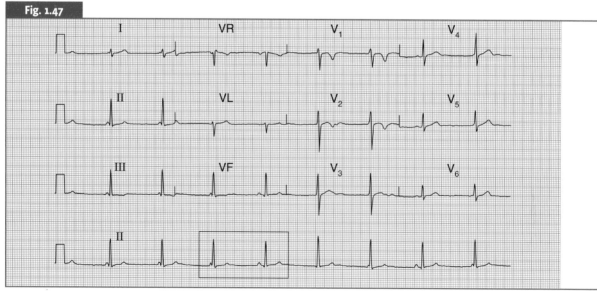

Fig. 1.47

Normal ECG
NOTE
- Very large U waves following normal T waves in leads V_1–V_4

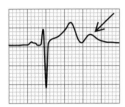

Very large U wave in lead V_3

Normal ECG with accelerated idionodal rhythm
NOTE
- SA node stimulates the atria at a constant rate of 50 bpm
- Ventricular rate is slightly faster than the atrial rate
- Narrow QRS complexes, originating in the AV node
- QRS complexes appear to 'overtake' the P waves, which are not suppressed – causing an apparent variation in the PR interval

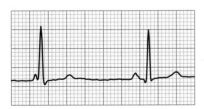

Variation of PR interval

The ECG in athletes

Any of the normal variations discussed above can be found in athletes. There can be changes in rhythm and/ or ECG pattern, and the ECGs of athletes may also show some features that might be considered abnormal in non-athletic subjects, but are normal in athletes (see Box 1.5). Fig. 1.47 shows the short and varying PR interval of an 'accelerated idionodal rhythm' (also known as a 'wandering atrial pacemaker'). Here the sinus node rate has slowed, and the heart rate is controlled by the AV node, which is discharging faster than the sinoatrial (SA) node.

The ECGs in Figs 1.47–1.49 were all recorded during the screening examinations of healthy young footballers.

BOX 1.5 Possible ECG Features of Healthy Athletes

Variations in Rhythm
- Sinus bradycardia
- Marked sinus arrhythmia
- Junctional rhythm
- 'Wandering' atrial pacemaker
- First degree block
- Wenckebach phenomenon
- Second degree block

Variations in ECG Pattern
- Tall P waves
- Prominent septal Q waves
- Tall R waves and deep S waves
- Counterclockwise rotation
- Slight ST segment elevation
- Tall symmetrical T waves
- T-wave inversion, especially in lateral leads
- Biphasic T waves
- Prominent U waves

Fig. 1.48

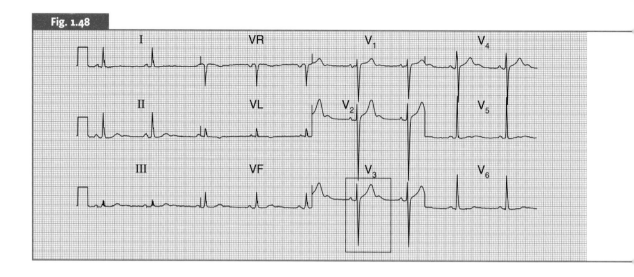

Fig. 1.49

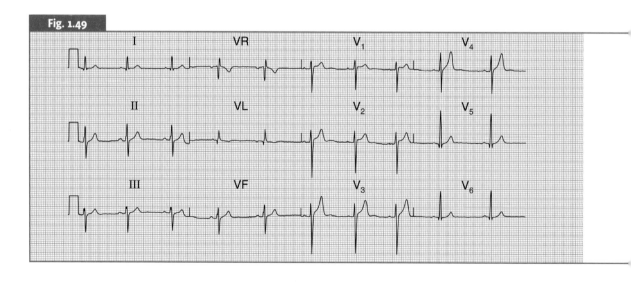

Normal ECG

NOTE

- Heart rate 53 bpm
- Sinus rhythm
- Prominent U waves in leads V_2–V_5
- Inverted T waves in lead VL

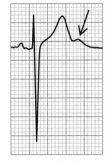

U wave in lead V_3

Normal ECG

NOTE

- Sinus rhythm
- Left axis deviation
- Septal Q waves in leads V_5–V_6

Fig. 1.50

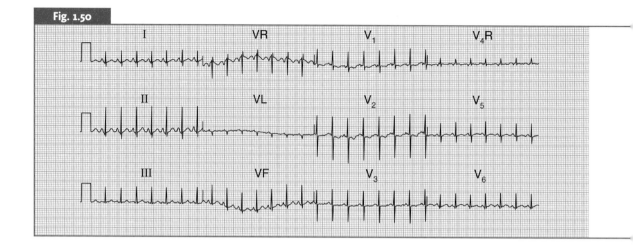

The ECG in pregnancy

Minor changes in the ECG are commonly seen in pregnancy (see Box 1.6). Ventricular extrasystoles are almost universal.

The ECG in children

The normal heart rate in the first year of life is 140–160 bpm, falling slowly to about 80 bpm by puberty. Sinus arrhythmia is usually quite marked in children.

At birth, the muscle of the right ventricle is as thick as that of the left ventricle. The ECG of a normal child in the first year of life has a pattern that would indicate right ventricular hypertrophy in an adult. The ECG in Fig. 1.50 was recorded from a normal 1-month-old child.

The changes suggestive of right ventricular hypertrophy disappear during the first few years of life. All the features

BOX 1.6 Possible ECG Features in Pregnancy

- Sinus tachycardia
- Supraventricular and ventricular extrasystoles
- Nonspecific ST segment/T wave changes

other than the inverted T waves in leads V_1 and V_2 should have disappeared by the age of 2 years, and the adult ECG pattern should have developed by the age of 10 years. In general, if the infant ECG pattern persists beyond the age of 2 years, then right ventricular hypertrophy is indeed present. If the normal adult pattern is present in the first year of life, then left ventricular hypertrophy is present.

The ECG changes associated with childhood are summarized in Box 1.7.

Normal ECG, from a 1-month-old child

NOTE

- Heart rate 170 bpm
- Sinus rhythm
- Normal axis
- Dominant R waves in lead V_1
- Inverted T waves in leads V_1–V_2
- Biphasic T waves in lead V_3
- Lead V_4R (a position on the chest equivalent to V_4, but on the right side) has been recorded instead of V_4

What is a 'normal ECG'

In this chapter we have emphasized the importance of clinical context in the interpretation of the ECG and looked at a range of ECG variants which can occur in healthy patients (see Box 1.8). There are also a range of ECG abnormalities which may occur in asymptomatic patients before the development of symptoms (e.g. the arrhythmic syndromes) or where symptoms are atypical

BOX 1.7 The ECG in Normal Children

At Birth
- Sinus tachycardia
- Right axis deviation
- Dominant R waves in lead V_1
- Deep S waves in lead V_6
- T waves inverted in leads V_1–V_4

At 1 Year of Age
- Sinus tachycardia
- Right axis deviation
- Dominant R waves in lead V_1
- T waves inverted in leads V_1–V_2

At 2 Years of Age
- Normal axis
- S waves greater than R waves in lead V_1
- T waves inverted in leads V_1–V_2

At 5 Years of Age
- Normal QRS complexes
- T waves still inverted in leads V_1–V_2

At 10 Years of Age
- Adult pattern

or absent (e.g. atrial fibrillation is a frequent incidental finding, or evidence of a 'silent' old myocardial infarction). These will be discussed in the coming chapters. Finally, there are some 'abnormalities' which increase in prevalence with age and probably represent early subclinical heart disease. These can be useful markers of cardiac risk, particularly on a population basis.

ECG findings of early stages of conduction disorders are a good example of how cumulative ECG changes have clinical importance, even in asymptomatic patients. First degree block (especially when the PR interval is only slightly prolonged) can be a normal variant but also increases in prevalence with age, although it has little effect on prognosis. Second and third degree block indicate more advanced heart disease and the prognosis is worse, although the congenital form of complete block is less serious than the acquired form in adults. Likewise, left anterior hemiblock has a good prognosis, as does RBBB. However, there is evidence that left bundle branch block (LBBB), even in the absence of other manifestations of cardiac disease, is associated with an adverse prognosis compared with that of individuals with a normal ECG. The risk is worse if a subject known to have a normal ECG suddenly develops LBBB, even if there are no symptoms – the ECG change presumably indicates progressive cardiac disease, probably most often ischaemia. Bifascicular block seldom progresses to complete block, but is an indication of underlying heart disease – the prognosis is worse compared to that of patients with LBBB alone.

BOX 1.8 Variations in the Normal ECG in Adults

Rhythm
- Marked sinus arrhythmia, with escape beats
- Lack of sinus arrhythmia (normal with increasing age)
- Supraventricular extrasystoles
- Ventricular extrasystoles

P Wave
- Normally inverted in lead VR
- May be inverted in lead VL

Cardiac Axis
- Minor right axis deviation in tall people

QRS Complexes in the Chest Leads
- Slight dominance of R wave in lead V_1, provided there is no other evidence of right ventricular hypertrophy or posterior infarction
- The R wave in the lateral chest leads may exceed 25 mm in thin fit young people

- Partial right bundle branch block (RSR[1] pattern, with QRS complexes less than 120 ms)
- Septal Q waves in leads III, VL, V_5–V_6

ST Segment
- Raised in anterior leads following an S wave (high take-off ST segment)
- Depressed in pregnancy
- Nonspecific upward-sloping depression

T Wave
- Inverted in lead VR and often in V_1
- Inverted in leads V_2–V_3, or even V_4 in people of African origin
- May invert with hyperventilation
- Peaked, especially if the T waves are tall

U Wave
- Normal in anterior leads when the T wave is not flattened

WHAT TO DO

When an apparently asymptomatic subject has an ECG record that appears abnormal, the most important thing is not to cause unnecessary alarm. There are four questions to ask:

1. Does the ECG really come from that individual? If so, is he or she really asymptomatic and are the findings of the physical examination really normal (particularly in patients who may be too functionally limited to provoke symptoms)?
2. Is the ECG really abnormal or is it within the normal range?
3. If the ECG is indeed abnormal, what are the implications for the patient? Is it important?
4. What (if any) further investigations or treatments are needed?

Further investigations

Complex and expensive investigations are seldom justified in asymptomatic patients whose hearts are clinically normal, but who have been found to have an abnormal ECG. Where there is uncertainty, an assessment of cardiac structure and function (usually with an echocardiogram) is the most helpful investigation.

Table 1.1 shows investigations that should be considered in the case of various cardiac rhythms and indicates which underlying diseases may be present.

Treatment of asymptomatic ECG abnormalities

It is always the patient who should be treated, not the ECG, but there are some circumstances where treatment should be considered in asymptomatic patients. The prognosis of patients with higher degree AV block is improved by permanent pacing. Atrial fibrillation need not be treated if the ventricular rate is reasonable, but anticoagulation must be considered in accordance with current guidelines. Patients at high risk of occult ischaemic heart disease (IHD) should be considered for therapies to address risk factors such as diabetes, hypertension, and dyslipidaemia.

TABLE 1.1 Investigations in Apparently Healthy People With an Abnormal ECG

ECG appearance	Diagnosis to be excluded	Possible investigations
Sinus tachycardia	Thyrotoxicosis Anaemia Changes in heart size Heart failure Systolic dysfunction	Thyroid function Haemoglobin Echocardiogram
Sinus bradycardia	Myxoedema	Thyroid function
Frequent ventricular extrasystoles	Left ventricular dysfunction Anaemia	Echocardiogram Haemoglobin Investigations for IHD
Right bundle branch block	Heart size Lung disease Atrial septal defect	Echocardiogram
Left bundle branch block	Heart size Aortic stenosis Cardiomyopathy Ischaemia	Echocardiogram Investigations for IHD
T-wave abnormalities	High or low potassium or calcium Ventricular systolic dysfunction Hypertrophic cardiomyopathy Ischaemia	Electrolytes Echocardiogram Investigations for IHD

The ECG in patients with palpitations and syncope: initial assessment

2

The clinical history and physical examination	**57**
Palpitations	57
Dizziness and syncope	58
Physical examination	62
The ECG	**62**
Syncope due to cardiac disease other than arrhythmias	62
Patients with possible tachycardias	68
Patients with possible bradycardias	77

The ECG is of paramount importance for the diagnosis of arrhythmias. Many arrhythmias are not noticed by the patient, but are still of clinical importance (e.g. atrial fibrillation). Symptoms, when they occur, are often transient, and the patient may be completely well at the time he or she consults a doctor. A baseline 12-lead ECG is a critical element of the initial assessment of anyone with suspected arrhythmia, but as always the history and physical examination are also extremely important. The main purpose of the history and examination is to help decide whether a patient's symptoms could be the result of an arrhythmia, and whether the patient has a cardiac or other disease that may cause an arrhythmia.

THE CLINICAL HISTORY AND PHYSICAL EXAMINATION

Palpitations

'Palpitations' mean different things to different patients, but a general definition would be 'an awareness of the heartbeat'. Arrhythmias, fast or slow, can cause poor organ perfusion and so lead to syncope (a word used to describe all sorts of collapse), breathlessness and angina. Some rhythms can be identified from a patient's description, such as:

- A patient recognizes sinus tachycardia because it feels like the palpitations that he or she associates with anxiety or exercise.
- Extrasystoles are described as the heart 'jumping' or 'missing a beat'. It is not possible to distinguish between supraventricular and ventricular extrasystoles from a patient's description, although they can be differentiated from an ECG.
- A true pathological tachyarrhythmia such as an atrioventricular (AV) nodal re-entry tachycardia

TABLE 2.1 Diagnosis of Sinus Tachycardia or a Pathological Tachycardia From a Patient's Symptoms

Symptoms	Sinus tachycardia	Pathological tachycardia
Timing of initial attack	Attacks probably began recently	Attacks probably began in teens or early adult life
Associations of attack	Exercise, anxiety	Usually no associations, but occasionally exercise-induced
Rate of start of palpitations	Slow build-up	Sudden onset
Rate of end of palpitations	'Die away'	Classically sudden, but often 'die away'
Heart rate	< 140 bpm	> 160 bpm
Associated symptoms	Paraesthesia due to hyperventilation	Chest pain Breathlessness Dizziness Syncope
Ways of terminating attacks	Relaxation	Breath holding] in some arrhythmias Valsalva's manoeuvre]

begins suddenly and sometimes stops suddenly. The heart rate is often 'too fast to count'. Severe attacks are associated with dizziness, breathlessness and chest pain (Table 2.1).

Dizziness and syncope

These symptoms may have a cardiovascular or a neurological cause. Remember that cerebral hypoxia, however caused, may lead to a seizure, and that can make the differentiation between cardiac and neurological syncope very difficult. Syncope is defined as 'a transient loss of consciousness characterized by unresponsiveness and loss of postural tone, with spontaneous recovery and not requiring specific resuscitative intervention'.

Fig. 2.1 shows an EEG that was being recorded in a 46-year-old woman with episodes of limb shaking, suspected of being generalized tonic–clonic seizures. She lost awareness during events, and had violent limb shaking for several seconds as she came round. She felt nauseated, but was rapidly reoriented. By chance, she had one of her 'attacks' while her EEG was being recorded, and from the

ECG being routinely recorded in parallel, it became clear that the problem was not seizures, but periods of asystole – in this case lasting about 15 s. The numbered arrows in Fig. 2.1 mark significant features. The recording begins with a routine period of hyperventilation, with the EEG showing an eye-blink in the anterior leads and the ECG showing sinus rhythm. There are then (at arrow 1 on the record) one (or possibly two) ventricular extrasystoles, followed by a narrow complex beat (probably sinus) and another ventricular extrasystole, with a different configuration from the previous ones. Asystole follows, and after 7–8 s (at arrow 2) there is global EEG slowing, and the patient became unresponsive. After 4 s (at arrow 3), there is global attenuation (reduction in signals) in the EEG and after another 3 s, there is an escape beat whose morphology suggests a ventricular origin. This is followed by a beat with a narrow QRS complex and possibly an inverted T wave, and then there is gross artefact due to the ECG lead being checked. During that period, sinus rhythm was restored. There was then (at arrow 4) global EEG slowing for 5 s, followed by (at arrow 5) violent limb thrashing for about 12 s as the patient regained consciousness – these movements were not clonic, and were thought to represent anxiety or fear. Normal EEG and ECG activity were then resumed (at arrow 6).

Some causes of syncope are summarized in Box 2.1.

Table 2.2 shows some clinical features of syncope, and possible causes.

BOX 2.1 Cardiovascular Causes of Syncope

Obstructed blood flow in heart or lungs
- Aortic stenosis
- Pulmonary embolus
- Pulmonary hypertension
- Hypertrophic cardiomyopathy
- Pericardial tamponade
- Atrial myxoma

Arrhythmias
- Tachycardias: patient is usually aware of a fast heartbeat before becoming dizzy
- Bradycardias: slow heart rates are often not appreciated. A classical cause of syncope is a Stokes–Adams attack, due to a very slow ventricular rate in patients with complete heart block. A Stokes–Adams attack can be recognized because the patient is initially pale but flushes red on recovery

Postural hypotension, occurring immediately on standing
Seen with:
- Loss of blood volume
- Autonomic nervous system disease (e.g. diabetes, Shy–Drager syndrome, amyloid neuropathy)
- Patients being treated with antihypertensive drugs

Neurally mediated reflex syncopal syndromes
- Vasovagal (neurocardiogenic) (simple faints)
- Situational (e.g. after coughing, sneezing, gastrointestinal stimulation of various sorts, postmicturition)
- Carotid sinus hypersensitivity

TABLE 2.2 Diagnosis of Causes of Syncope

Symptoms and signs	Possible diagnosis
Family history of sudden death	Long QT syndrome, Brugada syndrome, hypertrophic cardiomyopathy
Caused by unpleasant stimuli, prolonged standing, hot places (situational syncope)	Vasovagal syncope
Occurs within seconds or minutes of standing	Orthostatic hypotension
Temporal relation to medication	Orthostatic hypotension
Occurs during exertion	Obstruction to blood flow (e.g. aortic stenosis, pulmonary hypertension)
Occurs with head rotation or pressure on neck	Carotid sinus hypersensitivity
Confusion for more than 5 min afterwards	Seizure
Tonic–clonic movements, automatism	Seizure
Frequent attacks, usually unobserved, with somatic symptoms	Psychiatric illness
Symptoms or signs suggesting cardiac disease	Cardiac disease

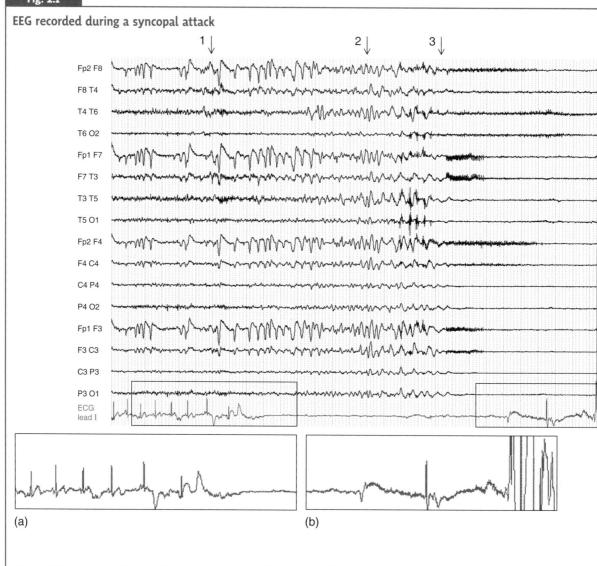

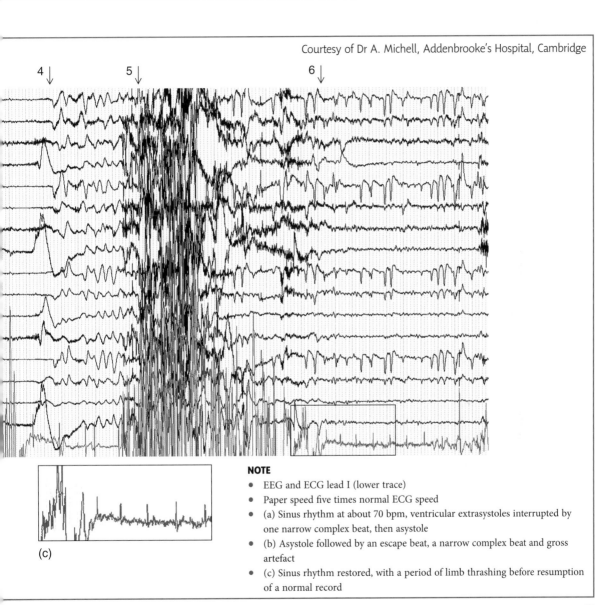

Courtesy of Dr A. Michell, Addenbrooke's Hospital, Cambridge

(c)

NOTE
- EEG and ECG lead I (lower trace)
- Paper speed five times normal ECG speed
- (a) Sinus rhythm at about 70 bpm, ventricular extrasystoles interrupted by one narrow complex beat, then asystole
- (b) Asystole followed by an escape beat, a narrow complex beat and gross artefact
- (c) Sinus rhythm restored, with a period of limb thrashing before resumption of a normal record

Physical examination

If the patient has no symptoms at the time of the examination, look for:

- evidence of any heart disease that might cause an arrhythmia
- evidence of non-cardiac disease that might cause an arrhythmia
- evidence of cardiovascular disease that might cause syncope without an arrhythmia
- evidence (from the history or examination) of neurological disease.

It is only possible to make a confident diagnosis that an arrhythmia is the cause of palpitations or syncope if an ECG recording of the arrhythmia can be obtained at the time of the patient's symptoms. If the patient is asymptomatic at the time of examination, it may be worth arranging for an ECG to be recorded during an attack of palpitations, or for a period of continuous 'ambulatory'

ECG monitoring (see Ch. 3), in the hope that an episode of the arrhythmia will be detected.

THE ECG

Even when the patient is asymptomatic, the resting 12-lead ECG can be very helpful, as summarized in Table 2.3.

Syncope due to cardiac disease other than arrhythmias

The ECG may indicate that syncopal attacks have a cardiovascular cause other than an arrhythmia.

ECG evidence of left ventricular hypertrophy or of left bundle branch block may suggest that syncope is due to aortic stenosis. The ECGs in Figs 2.2 and 2.3 were recorded from patients who had syncopal attacks on exercise due to severe aortic stenosis.

Fig. 2.2

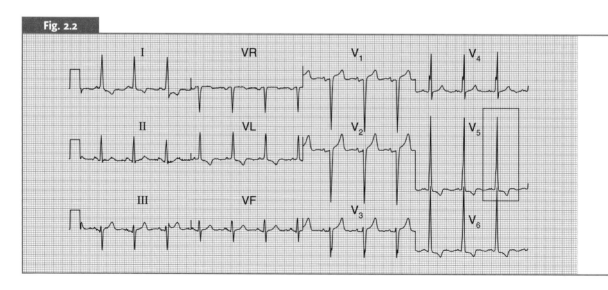

TABLE 2.3 ECG Features Between Attacks of Palpitations or Syncope

ECG appearance	Possible cause of symptoms
ECG completely normal	Symptoms may not be due to a primary arrhythmia – consider anxiety, epilepsy, atrial myxoma or carotid sinus hypersensitivity
ECGs that suggest cardiac disease	Left ventricular hypertrophy or left bundle branch block – aortic stenosis Right ventricular hypertrophy – pulmonary hypertension Anterior T wave inversion – hypertrophic cardiomyopathy
ECGs that suggest intermittent tachyarrhythmia	Left atrial hypertrophy – mitral stenosis, so possibly atrial fibrillation Pre-excitation syndromes Long QT syndrome Flat T waves suggest hypokalaemia Digoxin effect – ?digoxin toxicity
ECGs that suggest intermittent bradyarrhythmia	Second degree block First degree block plus bundle branch block Digoxin effect

Left ventricular hypertrophy
NOTE

- Sinus rhythm
- Bifid P waves suggest left atrial hypertrophy (best seen in leads V_4–V_5)
- Normal axis
- Tall R waves and deep S waves
- T waves inverted in leads I, VL, V_5–V_6

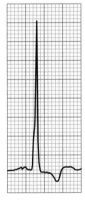

Tall R wave, inverted T wave in lead V_5

Fig. 2.3

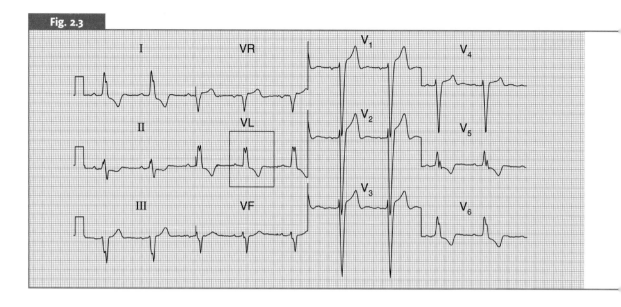

Fig. 2.4

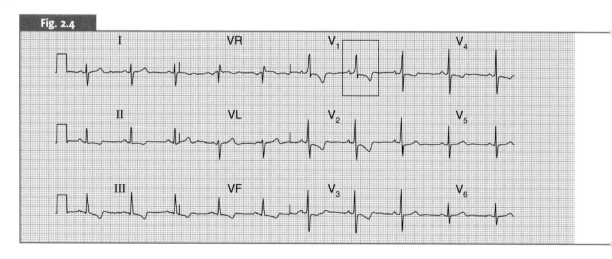

ECG evidence of right ventricular hypertrophy suggests thromboembolic pulmonary hypertension. The ECG in Fig. 2.4 is that of a middle-aged woman with dizziness on exertion, due to multiple pulmonary emboli.

Left bundle branch block
NOTE

- Sinus rhythm
- Slight PR interval prolongation (212 ms)
- Broad QRS complexes
- 'M' pattern in lateral leads
- T wave inversion in leads I, VL, V_5–V_6

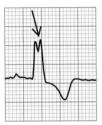

M pattern of left bundle branch block in lead VL

Right ventricular hypertrophy
NOTE

- Sinus rhythm
- Right axis deviation
- Dominant R waves in lead V_1
- Inverted T waves in leads V_1–V_4

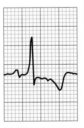

Dominant R wave in lead V_1

Fig. 2.5

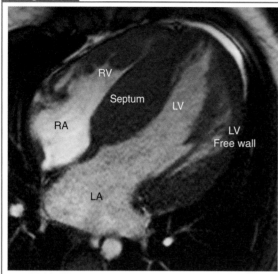

MR image of a heart with hypertrophic cardiomyopathy

NOTE

- RA – right atrium
- RV – right ventricular cavity
- Septum – interventricular septum (grossly hypertrophied)
- LV – left ventricular cavity
- LA – left atrium
- LV free wall – left ventricular myocardium

Fig. 2.6

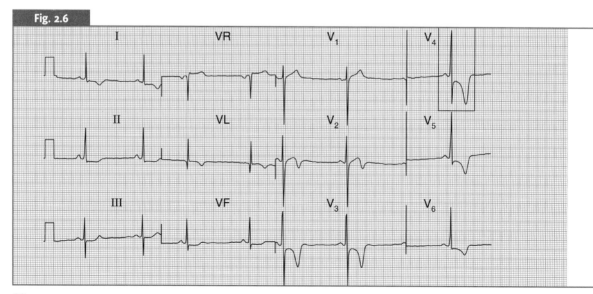

Syncope due to hypertrophic cardiomyopathy (HCM) (Fig. 2.5) may be associated with a characteristic ECG (Fig. 2.6) that resembles that of patients with an anterior non-ST elevation myocardial infarction (NSTEMI) (compare with Fig. 6.22, p. 222). With HCM, the T wave inversion is usually more pronounced than with an NSTEMI, and the R and S wave voltages may be increased (see page 21). HCM can cause syncope due to obstruction to outflow from the left ventricle, or can cause symptomatic angina or arrhythmias but not infrequently may be first identified through investigation of an ECG abnormality in a patient without typical symptoms. HCM is associated with an increased risk of atrial fibrillation as well as pathological arrhythmias. Genetic testing and family screening are recommended.

Hypertrophic cardiomyopathy

NOTE

- Sinus rhythm
- Marked T wave inversion in leads V_3–V_6

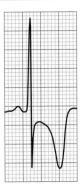

Inverted T wave in lead V_4

Patients with possible tachycardias
Mitral stenosis

Mitral stenosis leads to atrial fibrillation, but when the heart is still in sinus rhythm the presence of the characteristics of left atrial hypertrophy on the ECG may give a clue that paroxysmal atrial fibrillation is occurring (Fig. 2.7).

Pre-excitation syndromes

Normal conduction between the atria and ventricles involves the uniform spread of the depolarization wave front in a constant direction, down the bundle of His. In the pre-excitation syndromes, an abnormal additional pathway, or multiple pathways, connects the atria and ventricles. These accessory pathways bypass the AV node, where normal conduction is delayed, and therefore conduct more rapidly than the normal pathway. The anatomical combination of the normal AV node–His bundle pathway and the accessory pathway creates a potential circuit around which excitation may spread, causing a 're-entry' tachycardia (Ch. 4, p. 98).

The Wolff–Parkinson–White Syndrome

In the Wolff–Parkinson–White (WPW) syndrome, an accessory pathway (the 'bundle of Kent') connects either the left

Fig. 2.7

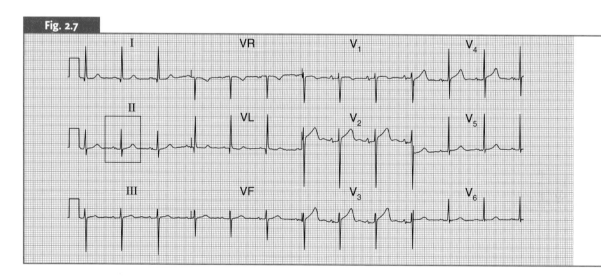

atrium and left ventricle, or the right atrium and right ventricle. Antegrade (from atrium to ventricle) conduction when in sinus rhythm in some cases may occur only through the normal His bundle pathway, so the QRS complexes will be normal and narrow; the accessory pathway is then said to be 'concealed'. In other 'manifest' cases, conduction may occur through both pathways simultaneously, but the heart will remain in sinus rhythm if conduction occurs in a forward direction (from atria to ventricles only) via both the AV node–His bundle pathway and the accessory pathway. The faster conduction down the accessory pathway causes part of the ventricle to depolarize early, resulting in a short PR interval and a slurred upstroke to the QRS complex (delta wave), causing a wide QRS complex. In 'latent' cases, antegrade conduction is variable and changes on the baseline ECG may come and go. In these cases pharmacological AV nodal blockade with adenosine may unmask the accessory pathway.

With a left-sided accessory pathway, the ECG shows a dominant R wave in lead V_1. This is called the 'type A'

pattern (Fig. 2.8). This pattern can easily be mistaken for right ventricular hypertrophy, the differentiation being made by the presence or absence of a short PR interval.

The ECG in Fig. 2.9 is from a young man who complained of symptoms that sounded like paroxysmal tachycardia. His ECG shows the WPW syndrome type A, but it would be quite easy to miss the short PR interval unless the whole of the 12-lead trace were carefully inspected. The short PR interval and delta waves are most obvious in leads V_4 and V_5.

When the accessory pathway is on the right side of the heart, there is no dominant R wave in lead V_1, and this is called the 'type B' pattern (Fig. 2.10).

ECGs indicating pre-excitation of the WPW type are found in approximately 1 in every 3000 healthy young people. Only half of these ever have an episode of tachycardia, and many have only very occasional attacks.

The ECG features associated with the WPW syndrome are summarized in Box 2.2. A similar ECG with a short

---

Left atrial hypertrophy

NOTE

- Sinus rhythm
- Bifid P waves, most clearly seen in leads I, II, V_3–V_5

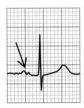

Bifid P wave in lead II

Fig. 2.8

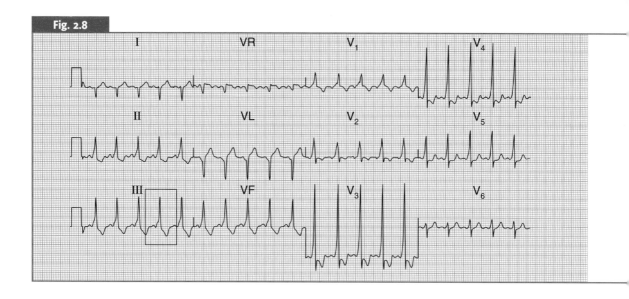

Fig. 2.9

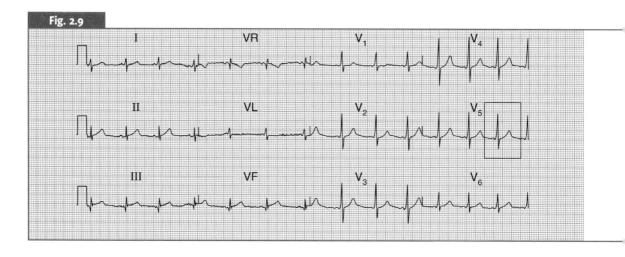

The Wolff–Parkinson–White syndrome, type A
NOTE

- Sinus rhythm
- Short PR interval
- Broad QRS complexes
- Dominant R wave in lead V_1
- Slurred upstroke to QRS complexes – the delta wave
- Inverted T waves in leads II, III, VF, V_1–V_4

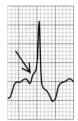

Delta wave in lead III

The Wolff–Parkinson–White syndrome, type A
NOTE

- Sinus rhythm
- Short PR interval, especially obvious in leads V_3–V_5
- Slurred upstroke to QRS complexes, obvious in leads V_3–V_5 but not obvious in the limb leads
- Dominant R wave in lead V_1
- No T wave inversion in the anterior leads (cf. Fig. 2.8)

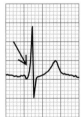

Delta wave in lead V_5

Fig. 2.10

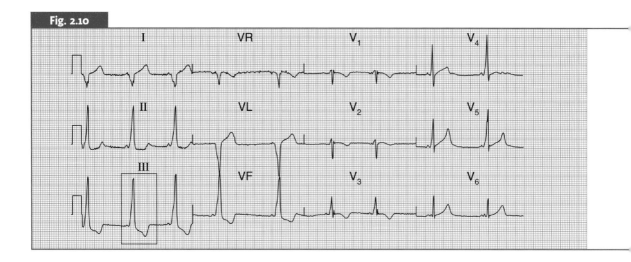

PR interval but with a normal QRS complex was previously referred to as the 'Lown–Ganong–Levine' syndrome although in the era of invasive cardiac electrophysiology, such distinctions have largely fallen out of use.

The long QT syndrome

Delayed repolarization occurs for a variety of reasons (Box 2.3) and causes a long QT interval. Assessment of the QT interval is discussed in Chapter 1 (page 47). A prolonged QT interval is associated with paroxysmal ventricular tachycardia and therefore can be the cause of episodes of collapse or even sudden death. The ventricular tachycardia associated with a prolonged QT interval usually involves a continual change from upright to downward QRS complexes. This is called 'torsade de pointes' (Fig. 2.11), and it usually occurs at times of increased sympathetic nervous system activity.

BOX 2.2 The Wolff–Parkinson–White Syndrome: ECG Features

- Short PR interval
- Wide QRS complexes with delta wave with normal terminal segment
- ST segment/T wave changes
- Left-sided pathway (type A): dominant R waves in leads V_1–V_6
- Right-sided pathway (type B): dominant S wave in lead V_1, and sometimes, anterior T wave inversion
- Arrhythmias (narrow or wide complex)
- Arrhythmia with wide, irregular complex suggests the WPW syndrome with atrial fibrillation

The Wolff–Parkinson–White syndrome, type B

NOTE

- Sinus rhythm
- Short PR interval
- Broad QRS complexes with delta waves
- No dominant R waves in lead V_1 (cf. Figs 2.8 and 2.9)
- T wave inversion in leads III, VF, V_3

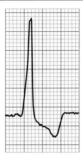

Short PR interval; broad QRS complex in lead III

Fig. 2.11

Torsade de pointes ventricular tachycardia

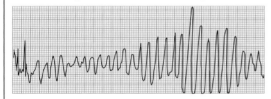

NOTE

- Broad complex tachycardia at 300 bpm
- Continually changing shape of QRS complexes

Several genetic abnormalities have been described that lead to familial prolongation of the QT interval and genetic family testing is recommended. The ECG in Fig. 2.12 is from a 10-year-old girl who suffered from 'fainting' attacks. Her sister had died suddenly; three other siblings and both parents had normal ECGs.

The most common cause of QT prolongation is drug therapy (Fig. 2.13 and Box 2.3).

Episodes of symptomatic ventricular tachycardia occur in about 8% of affected subjects each year, and the annual death rate due to arrhythmias is about 1% of patients with a long QT syndrome. The precise relationship between QT_C interval prolongation and the risk of sudden death is unknown; however, torsade de pointes ventricular tachycardia seems rare when the QT or QT_C interval is less than 500 ms.

Fig. 2.12

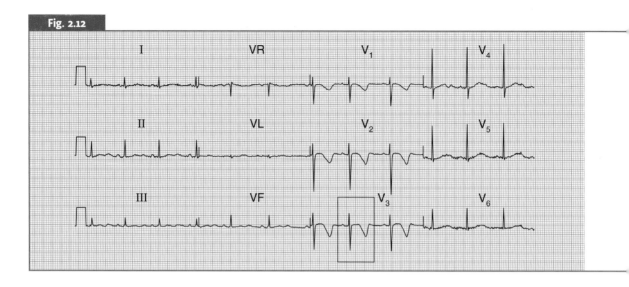

Fig. 2.13

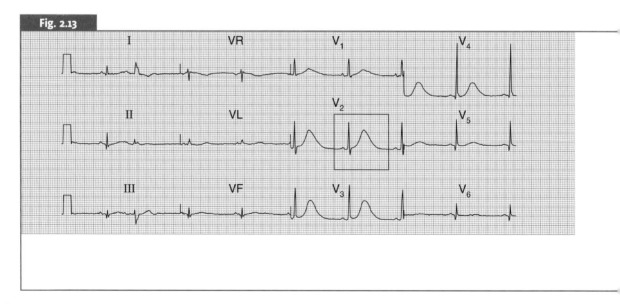

Congenital long QT syndrome

NOTE

- Sinus rhythm
- Normal axis
- QT interval 520 ms
- Marked T wave inversion in leads V_2–V_4

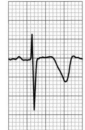

Long QT interval and inverted T wave in lead V_3

Prolonged QT interval due to amiodarone

NOTE

- Sinus rhythm
- Normal axis
- Dominant R waves in lead V_1 due to posterior infarction
- QT interval 800 ms
- Bizarre T wave shape in anterior leads

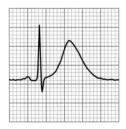

Long QT interval and bizarre T wave in lead V_2

BOX 2.3 Possible Causes of a Prolonged QT Interval

Congenital

- Jervell–Lange–Nielson syndrome; Romano–Ward syndrome

Antiarrhythmic drugs

- Amiodarone; Disopyramide; Flecainide; Procainamide; Propafenone; Quinidine (of historical interest only); Sotalol

Psychiatric drugs

- Amitriptyline; Chlorpromazine; Citalopram; Doxepin; Haloperidol; Imipramine; Lithium; Prochlorperazine; Risperidone

Antimicrobial, antifungal and antimalarial drugs

- Chloroquine; Clarithromycin; Co-trimoxazole (tri-methoprim–sulfamethoxazole); Erythromycin; Keto-conazole; Quinine

Antihistaminic drugs

- Fexofenadine

Other drugs

- Erythromycin; Tricyclic antidepressants

Plasma electrolyte abnormality

- Low potassium; Low magnesium; Low calcium

Others

- Alcohol; Tacrolimus; Tamoxifen

Note: There are many drugs which have been reported to cause prolongation of the QT interval. This is not an exhaustive list. See https://www.crediblemeds.org.

Fig. 2.14

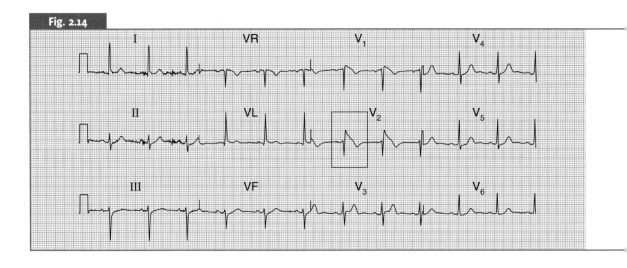

Fig. 2.15

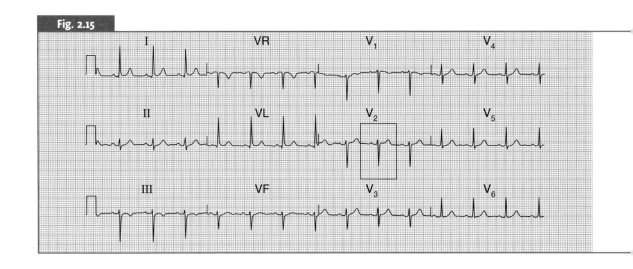

Brugada syndrome
NOTE
- Sinus rhythm
- Normal axis
- Normal QRS complex duration
- RSR^1 pattern in leads V$_1$–V$_2$
- No wide S wave in lead V$_6$
- Raised, downward-sloping ST segment in leads V$_1$–V$_2$

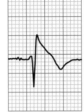

RSR^1 pattern and raised ST segment in lead V$_2$

Brugada syndrome
NOTE
- Same patient as in Fig. 2.14
- Normal ECG

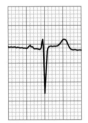

Normal appearance in lead V$_2$

The Brugada syndrome

Sudden collapse due to ventricular tachycardia and fibrillation occurs in a congenital disorder of sodium ion transport called the Brugada syndrome. Between attacks, the ECG superficially resembles that associated with right bundle branch block (RBBB), with an RSR^1 pattern in leads V$_1$ and V$_2$ (Fig. 2.14). However, the ST segment in these leads is raised, and there is no wide S wave in lead V$_6$ as there is in RBBB. The changes are seen in the right ventricular leads because the abnormal sodium channels are predominantly found in the right ventricle. The ECG abnormality can be transient – the ECG in Fig. 2.15 was taken a day later from the same patient as in Fig. 2.14. Pharmacological provocation testing is sometimes used to try to unmask the ECG features of Brugada syndrome where there is a clinical suspicion but the baseline ECG is not typical. Genetic and family screening are recommended and affected patients should avoid fever, alcohol and a number of drugs (see https://www.brugadadrugs.org).

Patients with possible bradycardias

When a patient is asymptomatic, an intermittent bradycardia can be suspected if the ECG shows any evidence of an escape rhythm or a conduction defect. However, it must be remembered that conduction defects and escape rhythms are quite common in healthy people, and their presence may be coincidental.

Escape rhythms

All myocardial cells will depolarize spontaneously if not stimulated by conduction of depolarization from neighbouring cells. This is called 'automaticity'. The automaticity of any part of the heart is suppressed by the arrival of a depolarization wave, and so the heart rate is controlled by the region with the highest automatic depolarization frequency. Normally the SA node controls the heart rate because it has the highest frequency of discharge, but if for any reason this fails, the region with the next highest intrinsic depolarization frequency will emerge as the pacemaker and set up an 'escape' rhythm. The atria and the junctional region have automatic depolarization frequencies of about 50 bpm, compared with the normal SA node frequency of 60–70 bpm. If both the SA node and the junctional region fail to depolarize, or if conduction to the ventricles fails, a ventricular focus may emerge, with a rate of 30–40 bpm; this is classically seen in complete heart block.

Escape beats may be single or may form sustained rhythms. They have the same ECG appearance as the corresponding extrasystoles, but appear late rather than early (Fig. 2.16).

In sustained junctional escape rhythms, atrial activation may be seen as a P wave following the QRS complex (Fig. 2.17). This occurs if depolarization spreads in the opposite direction from normal, from the AV node to the atria, and is called 'retrograde' conduction. Fig. 2.18 also shows a junctional escape rhythm.

Fig. 2.19 shows a ventricular escape beat.

Syncope

In a patient with syncopal attacks, ECG changes that would be ignored in a healthy person take on a greater significance. First degree block, itself of no clinical importance, may point to intermittent higher degree AV block (see Ch. 5).

Potentially significant conduction abnormalities. ECG evidence of AV conduction abnormalities will not be associated with syncope unless there is intermittent second or third degree heart block with a bradycardia. It is, however,

---

Fig. 2.16

Junctional escape beat

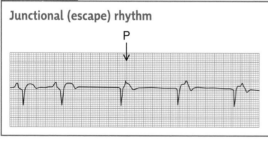

NOTE
- After two sinus beats there is no P wave
- After an interval there is a narrow QRS complex, with the same configuration as that of the sinus beats but without a preceding P wave
- This is a junctional beat (arrowed)
- Sinus rhythm then reappears

Fig. 2.17

Junctional (escape) rhythm

P

NOTE
- Two sinus beats are followed by an interval with no P waves
- A junctional rhythm then emerges (with QRS complexes the same as in sinus rhythm)
- A P wave (arrowed) can be seen as a hump on the T wave of the junctional beats: the atria have been depolarized retrogradely

important to recognize the presence of conduction defects because they may be pointers to intermittent heart block as a cause of syncopal attacks.

When first degree block is associated with left bundle branch block (Fig. 2.20), conduction must be delayed in either the AV node, the His bundle or the right bundle branch as well as in the left bundle branch. The combination of first degree block and RBBB (Fig. 2.21) shows that conduction has failed in the right bundle branch and is also beginning to fail elsewhere.

A combination of left anterior hemiblock and RBBB means that conduction into the ventricles is only passing through the posterior fascicle of the left bundle branch (Fig. 2.22). This is called 'bifascicular block'.

A combination of left anterior hemiblock, RBBB and first degree block suggests that there is disease in the remaining conducting pathway – either in the main His bundle or in the posterior fascicle of the left bundle branch. This is sometimes called 'trifascicular block' (Fig. 2.23). Complete conduction block in the right bundle and in both fascicles of the left bundle would, of course, cause complete (third degree) heart block, and intermittent left and right bundle branch block occurring in the same patient is associated with a high risk of higher degree AV block.

Fig. 2.18

Junctional (escape) rhythm

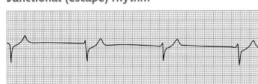

NOTE
- No P waves
- Narrow QRS complexes and normal T waves

Fig. 2.19

Ventricular escape beat

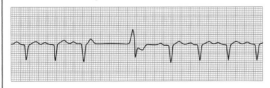

NOTE
- Three sinus beats are followed by a pause
- There is then a single ventricular beat with a wide QRS complex and an inverted T wave
- Sinus rhythm is then restored

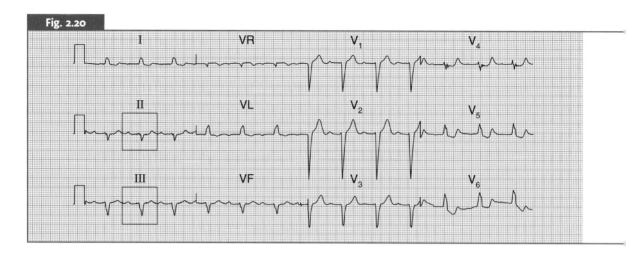

Fig. 2.20

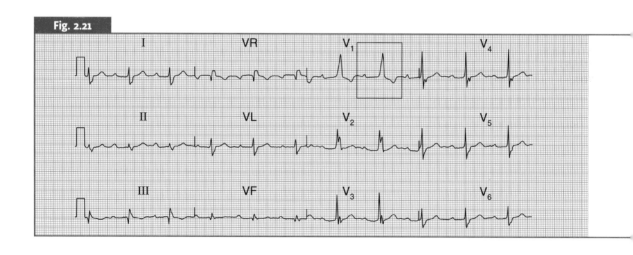

Fig. 2.21

First degree block and left bundle branch block (LBBB)

NOTE

- Sinus rhythm
- PR interval 300 ms
- LBBB pattern
- Broad QRS complexes

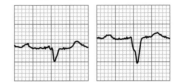

Long PR interval in leads II and III

First degree block and right bundle branch block (RBBB)

NOTE

- Sinus rhythm
- PR interval 328 ms
- Right axis deviation
- Broad QRS complexes
- RBBB pattern

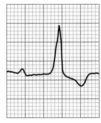

Long PR interval and RBBB pattern in lead V_1

Fig. 2.22

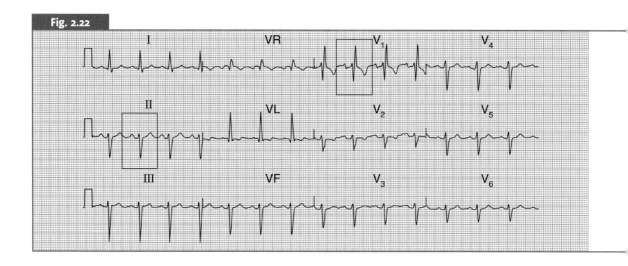

Fig. 2.23

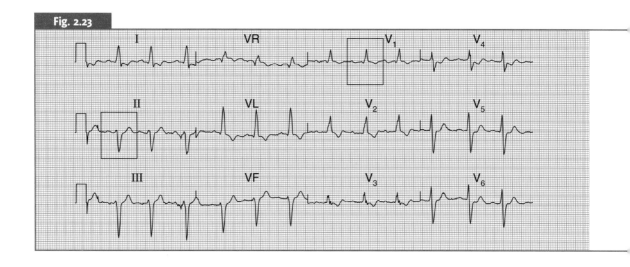

Bifascicular block

NOTE

- Sinus rhythm
- PR interval normal (176 ms)
- Left anterior hemiblock
- RBBB

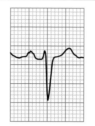 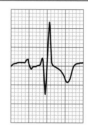

Left axis deviation and broad QRS complex in lead II

RBBB in lead V$_1$

Trifascicular block

NOTE

- Sinus rhythm
- PR interval 224 ms
- Left anterior hemiblock
- RBBB

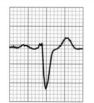 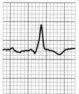

Left axis deviation in lead II

RBBB in lead V$_1$

The ECG in patients with palpitations and syncope: ambulatory ECG monitoring

3

Types of ECG monitors	85
Features of ambulatory ECG traces	86

Although sometimes a baseline ECG between episodes can provide supporting evidence for a potential diagnosis, the only way to be certain that a patient's symptoms are due to an arrhythmia is to show that an arrhythmia is present at the time of the symptoms. This may require ECG monitoring for longer periods than the 12-lead ECG, and in this chapter we will describe some of the technological options available for ambulatory monitoring of the ECG.

TYPES OF ECG MONITORS

There is an expanding range of ECG monitoring technologies available to aid diagnosis (Tables 3.1 and 3.2). Selecting the best options depends on local availability and the nature and frequency of patient episodes. If symptoms occur frequently – say two or three times a week – a 24- to 72-h tape recording (called a 'Holter' record after its inventor) may show the abnormality. Traditional lead-based monitors (Table 3.1a) are being replaced by disposable patch adhesive monitors (Table 3.2b) which are water

resistant to allow the patient to shower. These will often enable monitoring for a week or more if longer periods are needed. The latest wireless enabled devices can send data to a small device or hub, which can then relay data via the mobile phone network to the analytical centre for assessment.

If symptoms, although transient, are sustained over a longer period, a patient-activated Cardiac memo would traditionally be used (Table 3.1b). However, mobile phone-based ECG apps are becoming increasingly cost-effective. For example, electrodes mounted by adhesive onto a suitable mobile phone onto which the app has been enabled can be used to generate an ECG by simply placing one or more fingers from one hand onto one electrode and doing the same with the opposite hand onto the other electrode. The ECG traces can then be stored or relayed to the medical team for review with automated analytical functions also available (Table 3.2a).

When symptoms are infrequent, of short duration or lead to altered consciousness, 'event recorders' are more useful. These can either be patient-activated or programmed to record automatically an ECG in response to changes in detected heart rate or rhythm. External lead-based loop recorders (Table 3.1c) are again being superseded by patch or garment-mounted devices to improve patient convenience and compliance.

For longer periods of monitoring, implantable loop recorders can be used. These have reduced substantially in size (Table 3.1d and Table 3.2d) and can now be 'injected' through a very small incision. Again, patient activation (using an activator applied to the skin over the device) or automated rhythm detection allows ECGs of potential interest to be stored for subsequent analysis. Modern devices can relay data wirelessly which can then be sent via the mobile phone network to the medical team for review.

Table 3.1 shows traditional ECG monitoring devices and Table 3.2 shows newer available technologies.

FEATURES OF AMBULATORY ECG TRACES

Because of the limited number of vectors (due to the smaller number of electrodes used), ambulatory ECG monitors usually have fewer channels (sometimes just a single channel). Unlike the 12-lead ECG, which is usually taken at rest (except during formal exercise testing), ambulatory monitoring traces are more vulnerable to artefact due to motion. This can occasionally be misinterpreted as arrhythmia and should be considered when reviewing all such traces (Fig. 3.1).

Fig. 3.1

Movement artefact misinterpreted as a paroxysmal atrial fibrillation (boxed)

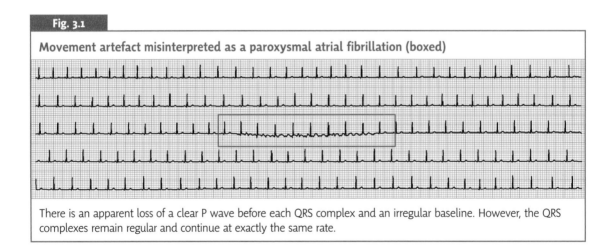

There is an apparent loss of a clear P wave before each QRS complex and an irregular baseline. However, the QRS complexes remain regular and continue at exactly the same rate.

Caution is also required to ensure asymptomatic arrhythmias are not over-interpreted as some rhythm variations are perfectly normal (see Ch. 1). For example, when 24-h recordings are made from healthy volunteers, extrasystoles are found in about two-thirds of them, and a few will even show the R on T phenomenon. Episodes of short runs of supraventricular tachycardia are seen in about 3% of apparently healthy subjects, and ventricular tachycardia in about 1%. As always, findings should be interpreted in the clinical context in which they are taken.

Figs 3.2 and 3.3 show examples of ambulatory records obtained from patients who complained of syncopal attacks, but whose hearts were in sinus rhythm at the time they were first seen.

Fig. 3.2

Trace from an implantable look recorder showing a sinus pause

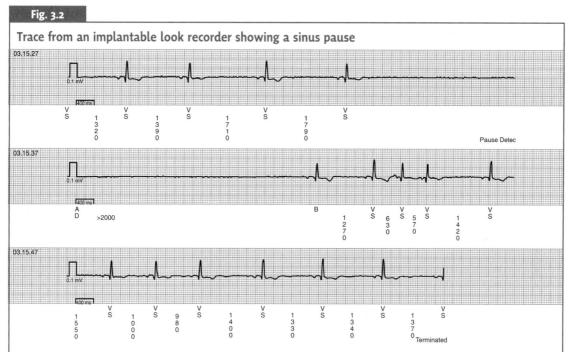

Below the single lead ECG trace, the automated rhythm analysis software detects each QRS complex (VS = ventricular sensing) and measures the R–R interval (the number recorded between each VS detected). The device correctly identifies an abnormality (AD), and the rhythm strip is saved and relayed for analysis.

TABLE 3.1 Traditional Ambulatory Cardiac Monitoring Devices

Monitoring device		Mode of use
(a) Holter monitor		
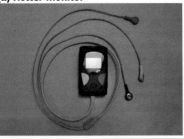	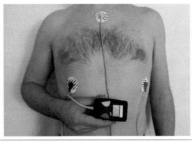	Usually three electrodes placed on chest wall for maximal signal; activation button can be used in association with patient diary to highlight symptomatic events
(b) Cardiac memo		
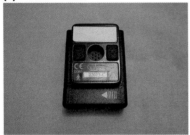	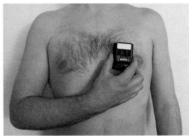	Device placed directly on to the skin by patient when symptomatic, or can be adapted to use with electrodes; traces can be downloaded by telephone
(c) Loop recorder		
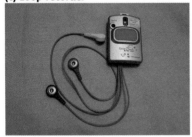	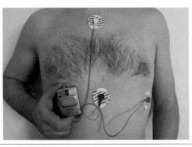	Usually three electrodes placed on chest wall; position of electrodes may require rotation, especially if there is skin reaction
(d) Implantable loop recorder		
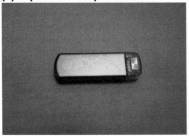	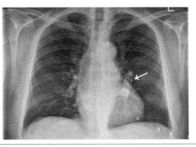	Requires subcutaneous implantation, a procedure taking around 20 min and with a low risk of infection Can be patient-activated

Duration and mode of recording	Applications	Comments
Usually 24 h, but up to 7 days Usually 1–2 channels, but up to 12 leads possible	Suitable for palpitations, syncope or presyncope occurring fairly frequently (e.g. daily)	Analysis time-consuming, but aided by software
10–20 recordings of 30–60 s	Suitable for palpitations lasting for several minutes, enabling patient to apply device and record trace	Not suitable for syncope, because patient activation required
Recording period programmable; usually 4 min pre-and post-activation Can record 2000–3000 periods ('loops') of ECG records, including patient-activated and autoactivated episodes Autoactivation function programmable, based on heart rate and on QRS complex duration and irregularity	Increasingly replacing memo devices Useful for diagnosis of palpitations or syncope	Can be kept in place for long periods, although batteries may need replacing periodically
Highly programmable; autoactivation can be based on heart rate and on QRS complex duration and irregularity	Especially useful for the diagnosis of rare rhythm disturbances and syncope	Orientation and site of implantation can be optimized prior to implantation Up to 14 months of battery life Surgical removal needed

TABLE 3.2 Newer Ambulatory Cardiac Monitoring Device Technology

Monitoring device	Mode of use
(a) Mobile phone apps	By placing a finger from opposite hands onto the mobile phone-mounted electrodes, the app can extract a rhythm strip for automated analysis

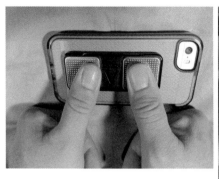 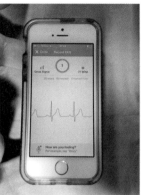 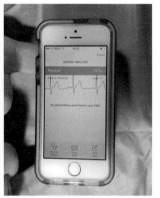

Monitoring device	Mode of use
(b) Patch ECG monitor	Direct application of the patch monitor to the skin allows continuous monitoring which can be relayed wirelessly to a hub and sent via the mobile phone network for analysis. Devices can be worn for many days and are water resistant

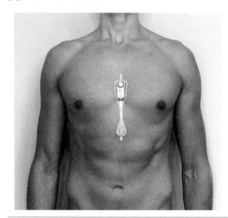

TABLE 3.2 Newer Ambulatory Cardiac Monitoring Device Technology—cont'd

Monitoring device	Mode of use
(c) Garment worn ECG monitor	Devices mounted in garments worn next to the skin can allow continuous ECG monitoring without the need for skin adhesives. Again the signal is wirelessly relayed to a hub and sent via the mobile phone network for analysis
(d) Mini loop recorder: mode of use 	As for the original implantable loop recorder but 'injected' through a much smaller puncture.

Fig. 3.3

Holter monitor trace showing initial sinus rhythm before a period of intermittent ventricular tachycardia

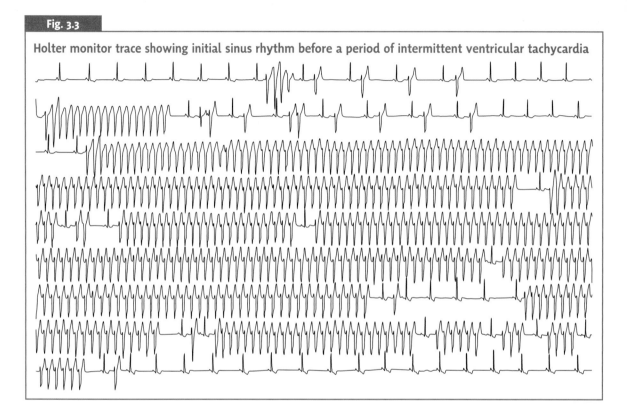

The ECG when the patient has a tachycardia

4

Mechanism of tachycardias	**93**
Enhanced automaticity and triggered activity	95
Abnormalities of cardiac rhythm due to re-entry	96
Differentiation between re-entry and enhanced automaticity	97
Extrasystoles causing symptoms	99
Narrow complex tachycardias causing symptoms	99
Broad complex tachycardias causing symptoms	113
Special forms of VT in patients with symptoms	131
Torsade de pointes	131
Broad complex tachycardia associated with the WPW syndrome	133
Management of arrhythmias	**133**
Electrophysiology and catheter ablation	**135**
The endocardial ECG	135
Catheter ablation	135
Arrhythmias amenable to ablation	138
Indications for electrophysiology	141
Cardiac arrest	**141**
ICD devices	141

The only tachycardia that can be (reasonably) reliably diagnosed from the patient's history is sinus tachycardia. A patient may notice the irregularity of atrial fibrillation, but it is easy to confuse this with multiple extrasystoles. The heart rate may give a clue to the nature of the arrhythmia (Table 4.1), but there is really no substitute for the ECG.

MECHANISM OF TACHYCARDIAS

Electrophysiology is the process of recording the ECG from inside the heart.

The main purpose of electrophysiological studies is to identify the site of origin of an arrhythmia. Arrhythmias occur either because of an abnormality of focal depolarization of the heart or because of re-entry circuits. If the origin can be localized, or the circuit disrupted, the arrhythmia may be prevented permanently by ablation. This technique uses local endocardial (or, more rarely, epicardial) cautery burns to abolish areas of abnormal cardiac electrical activity or to interrupt re-entry circuits.

TABLE 4.1 Physical Signs and Arrhythmias

Pulse	Heart rate (beats/min)	Possible nature of any arrhythmia
Arterial pulse		
Regular	< 50	Sinus bradycardia
		Second or third degree block
		Atrial flutter with 3:1 or 4:1 block
		Idionodal rhythm (junctional escape), with or without sick sinus syndrome
	60–140	Probable sinus rhythm
	140–160	Sinus tachycardia or an arrhythmia
	150	Probable atrial flutter with 2:1 block
	140–170	Atrial tachycardia
		Atrioventricular re-entry tachycardia (AVRT)
		Atrioventricular nodal re-entry tachycardia (AVNRT; junctional [nodal] tachycardia)
		Ventricular tachycardia
	> 180	Probable ventricular tachycardia
	300	Atrial flutter with 1:1 conduction
Irregular		Marked sinus arrhythmia
		Extrasystoles (supraventricular or ventricular)
		Atrial fibrillation
		Atrial flutter with variable block
		Rhythm varying between sinus rhythm and any arrhythmia or conduction defect
Jugular venous pulse		
More pulsations visible than heart rate		Second or third degree block
		Cannon waves – third degree block

Before the advent of electrical (ablation) therapy, the cause of arrhythmias was a fairly esoteric subject. Now, however, it is essential to understand the underlying electrical mechanisms, because they form the basis of ablation therapy.

Enhanced automaticity and triggered activity

If the intrinsic frequency of depolarization of the atrial, junctional or ventricular conducting tissue is increased, an abnormal rhythm may occur. This phenomenon is called 'enhanced automaticity'. Single early beats, or extrasystoles, may be due to enhanced automaticity arising from a myocardial focus. The most common example of a sustained rhythm due to enhanced automaticity is 'accelerated idioventricular rhythm', which is common after acute myocardial infarction. The ECG appearance (Fig. 4.1)

resembles that of a slow ventricular tachycardia (VT). This rhythm causes no symptoms and should not be treated.

If the junctional intrinsic frequency is increased to a point at which it approximates to that of the sinoatrial node, an 'accelerated idionodal rhythm' results. This may appear to 'overtake' the P waves (Fig. 4.2). This rhythm used to be called a 'wandering pacemaker'. Enhanced automaticity is also thought to be the mechanism causing some non-paroxysmal tachycardias, particularly those due to digoxin intoxication.

'Triggered activity' results from late depolarizations which occur after normal depolarization, during what would normally be a period of repolarization. Like enhanced automaticity, this can cause extrasystoles or a sustained arrhythmia, such as right ventricular outflow tract ventricular tachycardia (RVOT-VT) (Fig. 4.3).

Fig. 4.1

Accelerated idioventricular rhythm

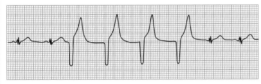

NOTE
- After two sinus beats, there are four beats of ventricular origin with a rate of 75 bpm
- Sinus rhythm is then restored

Fig. 4.2

Accelerated idionodal rhythm

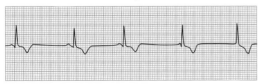

NOTE
- After three sinus beats, the sinus rate slows slightly
- A nodal rhythm appears and 'overtakes' the P waves

Fig. 4.3

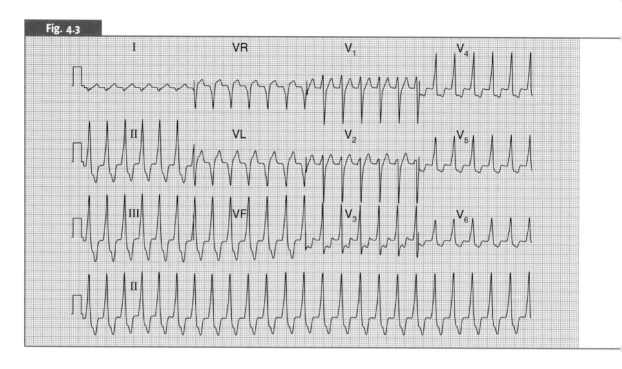

Abnormalities of cardiac rhythm due to re-entry

Normal conduction results in the uniform spread of the depolarization wave front in a constant direction. Should the direction of depolarization be reversed in some part of the heart, such as in an accessory connection between the atria and ventricles, it becomes possible for a circular or 're-entry' pathway to be set up. Activation travels round and round the circuit, causing a tachycardia such as the atrioventricular re-entry tachycardia (AVRT) experienced by patients with Wolff–Parkinson–White (WPW) syndrome or the atrioventricular nodal re-entry tachycardia (AVNRT) (Fig. 4.4).

Right ventricular outflow tract ventricular tachycardia (RVOT-VT)

NOTE

- Broad complex tachycardia
- Left bundle branch block and right axis deviation, typical of RVOT-VT

Differentiation between re-entry and enhanced automaticity

Except in the case of the pre-excitation syndromes, there is no certain way of distinguishing from the surface ECG between a tachycardia due to enhanced automaticity and one due to re-entry. In general, however, tachycardias that follow or are terminated by extrasystoles, and those that can be initiated or inhibited by appropriately timed intracardiac pacing impulses, are likely to be due to re-entry (Figs 4.5 and 4.6).

The differentiation between tachycardias caused by enhanced automaticity and those caused by re-entry does not affect the choice of drug treatment, and both can be treated by ablation.

Fig. 4.4

Re-entry pathways in the pre-excitation syndromes

AVRT

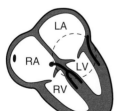

AVNRT

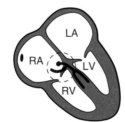

NOTE

- AVRT and AVNRT'

Fig. 4.5

Atrial tachycardia

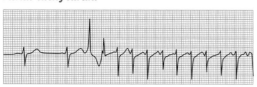

NOTE

- After two sinus beats there is one ventricular extrasystole, and then a narrow complex that is probably supraventricular
- Atrial tachycardia is induced
- P waves are visible at the end of the T wave of the preceding beat

Fig. 4.6

AV nodal re-entry tachycardia (AVNRT)

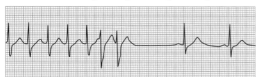

NOTE

- Five beats of AVNRT at 143 bpm are followed by two ventricular extrasystoles
- These interrupt the tachycardia, and sinus rhythm is restored

Fig. 4.7

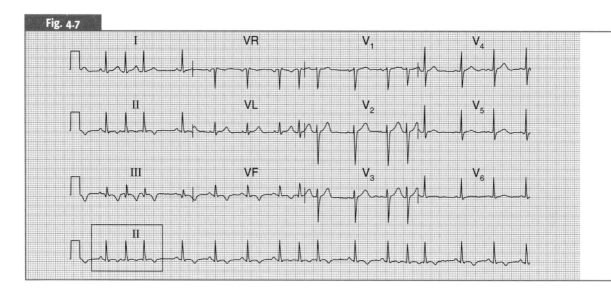

Extrasystoles causing symptoms

Occasional extrasystoles are a normal variant (see Ch. 1, p. 5, Figs 1.7 and 1.9). However, some patients may experience associated symptoms. Extrasystoles may occur in clusters. When occurring every other beat this is termed bigeminy, and when occurring every third beat trigeminy. Very frequent ventricular extrasystoles are sometimes associated with structural or ischaemic heart disease. An ECG is necessary to differentiate between supraventricular and ventricular extrasystoles.

When extrasystoles have a supraventricular origin (Fig. 4.7), the QRS complex is narrow and both it and the T wave have the same configuration as in the sinus beat. Atrial extrasystoles have abnormal P waves. Junctional (AV nodal) extrasystoles either have a P wave very close to the QRS complex (in front of it or behind it) or have no visible P waves.

Ventricular extrasystoles produce wide QRS complexes of abnormal shape, and the T wave is also usually abnormal. No P waves are present (Fig. 4.8).

When a ventricular extrasystole appears on the upstroke of the preceding beat, the 'R on T' phenomenon is said to be present (Fig. 4.9). This can initiate ventricular fibrillation, but usually it does not do so.

Narrow complex tachycardias causing symptoms

A tachycardia can be described as 'narrow complex' if the QRS complex is of normal duration, i.e. < 120 ms. Sinus and atrial arrhythmias as well as AVRT and AVNRT are all supraventricular. All these supraventricular rhythms have QRS complexes of normal shape and width, and the T waves have the same shape as in the sinus beat.

The types of narrow complex tachycardias are listed in Box 4.1.

Supraventricular extrasystoles

NOTE

- Sinus rhythm with atrial and junctional extrasystoles
- Normal axis
- Normal QRS complexes
- Inverted T waves in leads III, VF
- First beat: normal; second beat: atrial extrasystole, with abnormal P wave; third beat: AV nodal (junctional) extrasystole, with no P wave

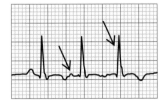

BOX 4.1 Narrow Complex Tachycardias

A regular narrow complex tachycardia may be:
- Sinus rhythm
- Atrial tachycardia
- Atrial flutter
- AV nodal re-entry tachycardia (AVNRT) – the most common type of supraventricular tachycardia
- AV re-entry tachycardia (AVRT), caused by the Wolff–Parkinson–White (WPW) syndrome with orthodromic conduction through the AV node–His bundle pathway

An irregular narrow complex tachycardia is usually:
- Atrial fibrillation

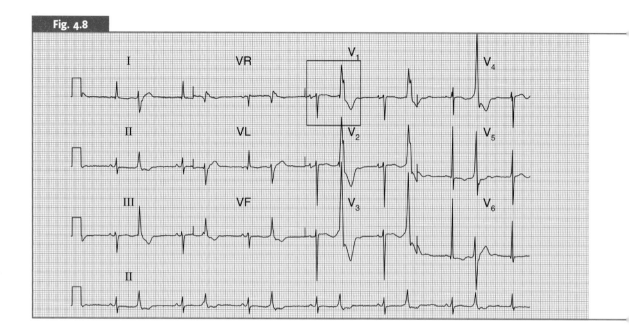

Fig. 4.8

Atrioventricular re-entry tachycardia

In the pre-excitation syndromes, normal and accessory pathways between an atrium and a ventricle together form an anatomical circuit around which depolarization can reverberate, causing a 're-entry' tachycardia (Fig. 4.10). Once established, a circular wave of depolarization will continue until some part of the pathway fails to conduct. Alternatively, the circular wave may be interrupted by the arrival of another depolarization wave, set up by an ectopic focus (e.g. an extrasystole).

In the WPW syndrome, the re-entry circuit comprises the normal AV node–His bundle connection between the atria and the ventricles, and an accessory pathway, the bundle of Kent, which also connects the atria and ventricles, bypassing the AV node (Fig. 4.4). If forward conduction in the accessory pathway is blocked (e.g. by an extrasystole causing the pathway to be transiently refractory to depolarization), conduction can spread down the normal pathway and back (i.e. retrogradely) via the accessory pathway (which by this time is no longer refractory), to reactivate the atria. Recurrent activation of the circuit can cause rapid cycling leading to a tachyarrhythmia.

Ventricular extrasystoles ('bigeminy')

NOTE

- Sinus rhythm with coupled ventricular extrasystoles
- Sinus beats show tall R waves and inverted T waves in leads V_5–V_6 (indicating left ventricular hypertrophy)
- Extrasystoles are of right bundle branch block (RBBB) configuration, and their T-wave inversion has no other significance

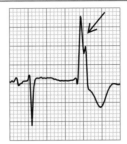

Extrasystole with RBBB configuration in lead V_1

Fig. 4.9

R on T phenomenon

NOTE

- Ventricular extrasystoles occurring near the peak of the preceding T wave

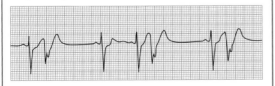

Fig. 4.10

Re-entry mechanisms causing tachycardia

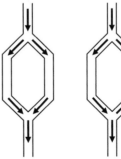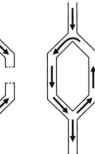

Normal   Conduction delay   Re-entry

Fig. 4.11

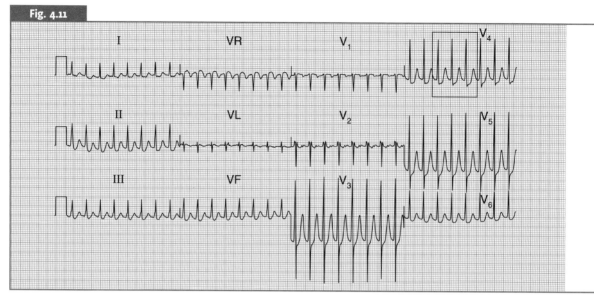

Fig. 4.12

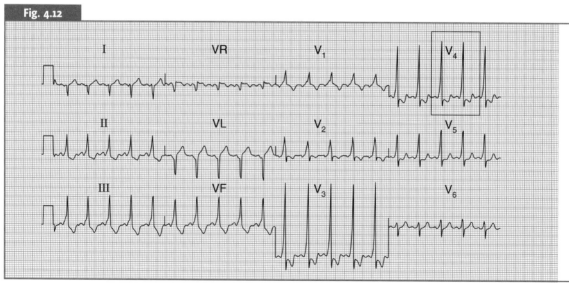

The tachycardia is described as 'orthodromic' when conduction within the His bundle is in the normal direction: the ECG then has narrow QRS complexes, and sometimes P waves are visible just after each QRS complex. The pattern resembles an AV nodal re-entry tachycardia (see below), and the presence of a pre-excitation syndrome may not be suspected until sinus rhythm is restored (Figs 4.11 and 4.12) – except in 'concealed cases' where the sinus 12-lead ECG may be normal (see Ch. 2, pp 68–72)

Less commonly, depolarization passes down the accessory pathway and retrogradely up the His bundle, to cause an 'antidromic reciprocating tachycardia', in which the QRS complexes are broad and slurred, and P waves may or may not be seen.

This is described below in the section on broad complex tachycardias (see page 135)

Supraventricular tachycardia

NOTE

- Narrow complex tachycardia
- No P waves visible
- Some ST segment depression, suggesting ischaemia

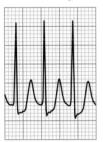

Narrow complexes with ST segment depression in lead V$_4$

Sinus rhythm, the Wolff–Parkinson–White syndrome, type A

NOTE

- Same patient as in Fig. 4.11, after cardioversion
- Sinus rhythm
- Short PR interval
- Broad QRS complexes with delta wave
- Dominant R wave in lead V$_1$ shows the WPW syndrome type A

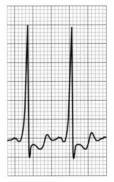

Short PR interval and delta wave in lead V$_4$

Fig. 4.13

AV nodal re-entry tachycardia (AVNRT)

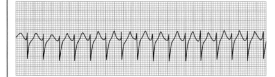

NOTE

- No P waves can be seen
- QRS complexes are narrow, and completely regular at 165 bpm

Fig. 4.14

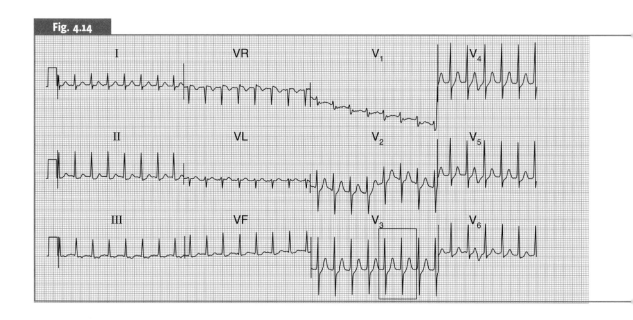

AV nodal re-entry tachycardia (AVNRT)

AVNRT, or junctional tachycardia, originates in or very close to the AV node or His bundle. It may be facilitated by a congenital abnormality of the AV node, in which there are two (or sometimes more) electrically distinct pathways. These allow re-entry to start and be sustained within the node itself. In the absence of a tachycardia, the sinus ECG has no distinguishing features, so the potential for

an AVNRT (as for a 'concealed' AVRT) cannot be detected from the baseline sinus ECG, unlike in cases of 'manifest' WPW. During AVNRT, atrial and ventricular activation are virtually simultaneous, so the P wave is hidden within the QRS complex (Figs 4.13 and 4.14). Carotid sinus pressure either reverts the heart to sinus rhythm or has no effect, but the circuit can usually be disrupted by administration of incremental doses of adenosine. The ECG in Fig. 4.14 shows a narrow complex tachycardia at 150 bpm, without any obvious P waves. After reversion to sinus rhythm (Fig. 4.15), the shape of the QRS complexes does not change.

Atrial tachycardia

Re-entry within the atrial muscle causes a tachycardia characterized by P waves with a different shape to those occurring with normal sinus beats. Atrial tachycardia can also result from enhanced automaticity. In atrial tachycardia (Fig. 4.16), P waves are present but they have an abnormal shape. They are sometimes hidden in the T wave of the preceding beat.

The P wave rate is in the range 130–250 bpm. When the atrial rate exceeds about 180 bpm, physiological block will occur in the AV node, so that the ventricular rate becomes half that of the atria.

Atrioventricular nodal re-entry tachycardia (AVNRT)

NOTE

- Regular narrow complex tachycardia, rate 150 bpm
- No P waves visible
- ST segment depression in leads II–III, VF suggests ischaemia

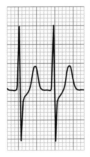

Narrow complexes at about 150 bpm in lead V_3

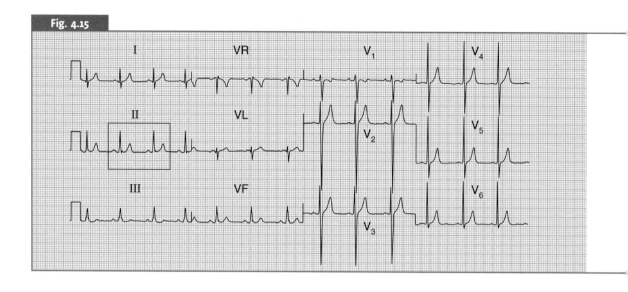

Fig. 4.15

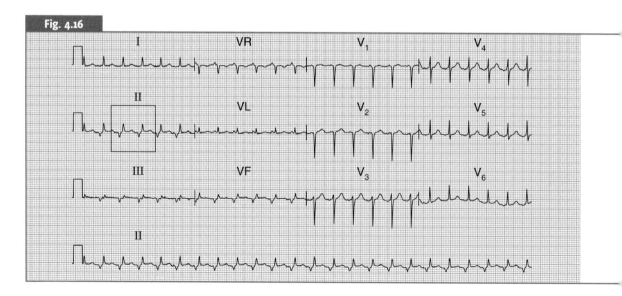

Fig. 4.16

Sinus rhythm following cardioversion

NOTE

- Same patient as in Fig. 4.14
- Sinus rhythm
- QRS complexes and T waves are the same shape as in AVNRT (Fig. 4.14)
- Now no suggestion of ischaemia

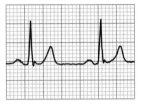

Sinus rhythm

Atrial tachycardia

NOTE

- Narrow complex tachycardia, heart rate 140 bpm
- Abnormally shaped P waves, one per QRS complex
- Short PR interval
- ECG otherwise normal

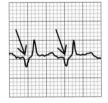

Abnormal P waves in lead II

Atrial flutter

Atrial flutter depends on a variety of re-entry circuits, which often occupy large areas of the atrium and are known as 'macro-re-entrant' circuits. The most common type of flutter, 'isthmus-dependent' flutter, involves circuits utilizing the cavotricuspid isthmus. The involvement of this defined isthmus is important in considering ablation therapy (see p. 139 and Fig. 4.48). In atrial flutter, the atrial rate is around 300 bpm and the P waves form a continuous 'sawtooth' pattern. As the AV node usually fails to conduct all the P waves, the relationship between P waves and QRS complexes is usually 2:1, 3:1 or 4:1. Fig. 4.17 shows atrial flutter with 2:1 block, giving a ventricular rate of 150 bpm. The ECG in Fig. 4.18 is from the same patient after reversion to sinus rhythm.

Fig. 4.17

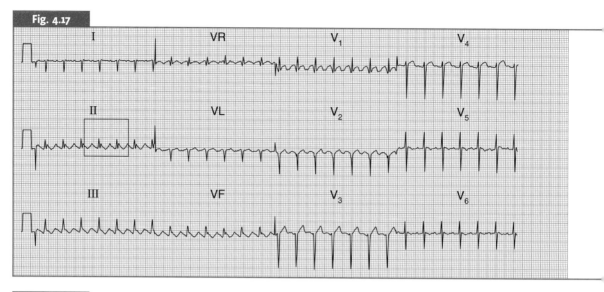

Fig. 4.18

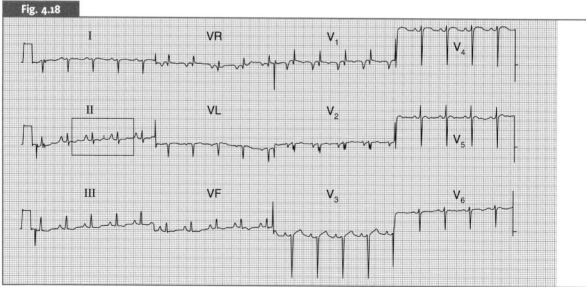

The ECG in Fig. 4.19 shows atrial flutter with 4:1 block.

The ECG in Fig. 4.20 shows a narrow complex (and therefore supraventricular) rhythm with a rate of 300 bpm. This is almost certainly atrial flutter with 1:1 conduction.

If the ventricular rate is rapid and P waves cannot be seen, carotid sinus pressure will usually increase the block in the AV node and make the 'sawtooth' more obvious.

Atrial flutter with 2:1 block

NOTE

- Regular narrow complex tachycardia
- 'Sawtooth' of atrial flutter most easily seen in lead II

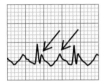

Flutter waves in lead II

Sinus rhythm, following cardioversion

NOTE

- Same patient as in Fig. 4.17
- Sinus rhythm
- Right axis deviation
- Dominant R waves in lead V_1
- Deep S waves in lead V_6, suggesting right ventricular hypertrophy
- The cardiac axis and QRS complexes have not been changed by cardioversion

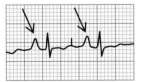

P waves in lead II

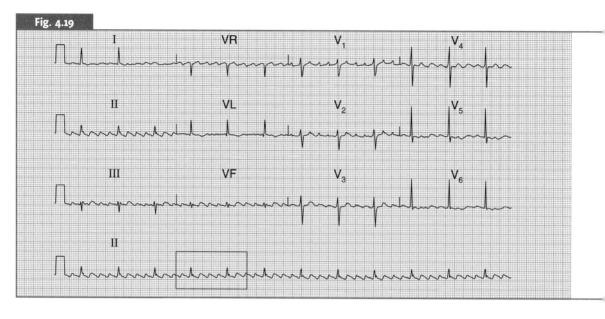

Fig. 4.19

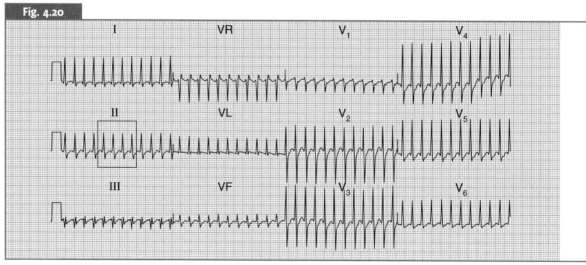

Fig. 4.20

Atrial flutter with 4:1 block

NOTE

- With 4:1 block and a ventricular rate of 72 bpm, flutter waves can be seen in all leads

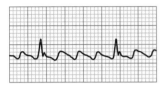

Flutter waves

Atrial flutter with 1:1 conduction

NOTE

- Narrow complex tachycardia at nearly 300 bpm
- No P waves visible
- Ventricular rate suggests that the underlying rhythm is atrial flutter

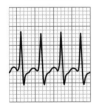

Narrow complex tachycardia at 300 bpm in lead II

Atrial fibrillation

In atrial fibrillation, disorganized atrial activity causes the P waves to disappear and the ECG baseline becomes totally irregular (Fig. 4.21). At times atrial activity may become sufficiently synchronized for a 'flutter-like' pattern to appear, but this rapidly breaks up (Fig. 4.22). In atrial fibrillation, as opposed to atrial flutter, the frequency of the QRS complexes is totally irregular.

Some causes of atrial fibrillation are summarized in Box 4.2.

> **BOX 4.2 Causes of Atrial Fibrillation (Paroxysmal or Persistent)**
>
> - Valvular (especially mitral) heart disease
> - Thyrotoxicosis
> - Alcoholism
> - Cardiomyopathy
> - Acute myocardial infarction
> - Chronic ischaemic heart disease
> - Hypertension
> - Myocarditis
> - Pericarditis
> - Pulmonary embolism
> - Pneumonia
> - Cardiac surgery
> - 'Lone' (i.e. no cause found)

Fig. 4.21

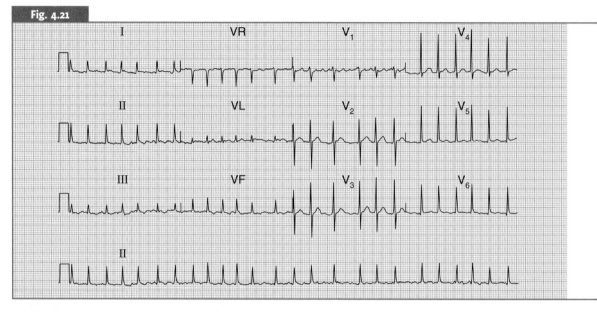

Fig. 4.22

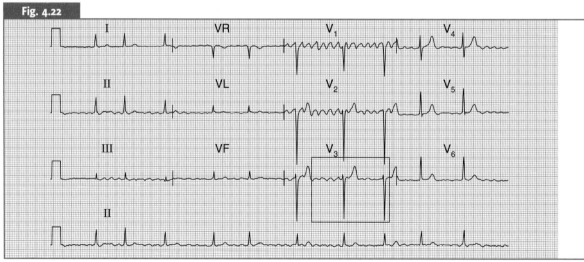

Atrial fibrillation

NOTE

- Irregular narrow complex tachycardia, 150 bpm
- During long R–R intervals, irregular baseline can be seen
- Suggestion of flutter waves in lead V_1

Atrial fibrillation

NOTE

- Irregular narrow complex rhythm
- Apparent flutter waves in lead V_1, but these are not constant, and from leads II and V_3 it is clear that this is atrial fibrillation

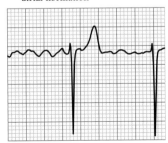

Atrial fibrillation

Broad complex tachycardias causing symptoms

'Broad complex' tachycardias are those in which the QRS complex duration exceeds 120 ms and which are not due to sinus rhythm with bundle branch block. Broad complex tachycardias can be either supraventricular with bundle branch block, or due to the WPW syndrome, or may be ventricular in origin. The types of broad complex tachycardia are listed in Box 4.3. Ventricular tachycardia (VT) may be due to re-entry through circuits within the ventricles (e.g. around areas of scar tissue following myocardial infarction), or may result from enhanced automaticity or triggered activity. The broad QRS complexes are of a constant configuration and are fairly regular if the re-entry pathway is constant (Fig. 4.23).

A supraventricular origin for a broad complex tachycardia can only be diagnosed with certainty when there is intermittent sinus rhythm with the same QRS complex configuration as is seen in the tachycardia (Fig. 4.24).

Here, we are concerned with broad complex rhythms without obvious P waves. These could be atrial fibrillation or junctional rhythms with bundle branch block, or could be ventricular rhythms. The differentiation of broad complex tachycardias can be difficult. It is not possible to distinguish between supraventricular and ventricular

---

BOX 4.3 Broad Complex Tachycardias

- Any supraventricular rhythm with bundle branch block
- Accelerated idioventricular rhythm (rate < 120 bpm)
- Ventricular tachycardia
- Torsade de pointes ventricular tachycardia
- The Wolff–Parkinson–White (WPW) syndrome

An irregular broad complex tachycardia is likely to be:
- Atrial fibrillation with bundle branch block
- Atrial fibrillation with the WPW syndrome

Fig. 4.23

Ventricular tachycardia

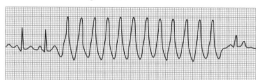

NOTE

- Two sinus beats are followed by ventricular tachycardia at 200 bpm
- The complexes are regular, with little variation in shape
- Sinus rhythm is then restored

Fig. 4.24

Junctional tachycardia with bundle branch block

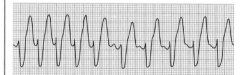

NOTE

- The first five beats show a broad QRS complex and there are no P waves
- Sinus rhythm is then restored and the QRS complex remains unchanged
- The tachycardia must be supraventricular with bundle branch block

Fig. 4.25

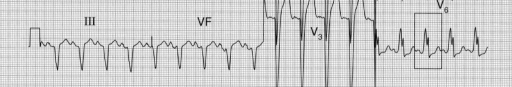
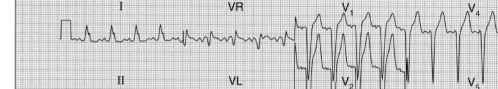

rhythms from the clinical state of the patient. Either type of rhythm can be well tolerated, and either can lead to cardiovascular collapse. However, broad complex tachycardias occurring in the course of an acute myocardial infarction (which is when they are most often seen) are almost always ventricular in origin. Other causes of VT are listed in Box 4.4.

With these things in mind, the ECG should be analysed logically. Look in turn for the following features:

1. The presence of P waves. If there is one P wave per QRS complex, it must be sinus rhythm with bundle branch block. If P waves can be seen at a slower rate than the QRS complexes, it must be VT.
2. QRS complex duration. If longer than 160 ms, it is probably VT.
3. QRS complex regularity. VT is usually regular. An irregular broad complex tachycardia usually means atrial fibrillation with abnormal conduction.
4. The cardiac axis. VT is usually associated with left axis deviation.

5. QRS complex configuration. If the QRS complexes in the V leads all point either upwards or downwards ('concordance'), it is probably VT.
6. When the QRS complex shows a right bundle branch block (RBBB) pattern, a supraventricular tachycardia with abnormal conduction is more likely if the second R peak is higher than the first. VT is likely if the first R peak is higher.
7. The presence of fusion and capture beats indicates that the broad complexes are due to VT (see p. 129).

P waves

The ECG in Fig. 4.25 is from a patient with an acute infarction, and shows a broad complex rhythm at about 110 bpm. One P wave per QRS complex can clearly be seen, and this is obviously sinus rhythm with left bundle branch block (LBBB).

Sinus rhythm with left bundle branch block (LBBB)

NOTE

- Sinus rhythm
- Left axis deviation
- Wide QRS complexes of LBBB configuration

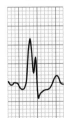

M wave of LBBB in lead V_6

BOX 4.4 Causes of Ventricular Tachycardia

- Acute myocardial infarction
- Chronic ischaemia
- Cardiomyopathy
  - hypertrophic
  - dilated
  - arrhythmogenic right ventricular cardiomyopathy
- Mitral valve prolapse
- Myocarditis
- Right ventricular outflow tract tachycardia
- Channelopathies (e.g. Brugada syndrome, long QT syndrome, cathecholaminergic polymorphic ventricular tachycardia)
- Electrolyte imbalance
- Drugs
  - antiarrhythmic
  - digoxin
- Idiopathic

Fig. 4.26

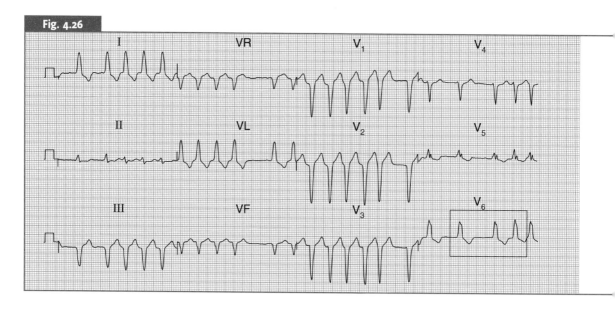

Fig. 4.27

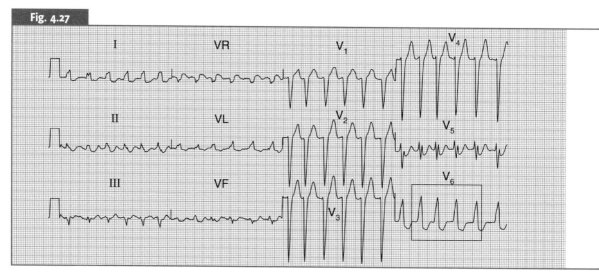

Atrial fibrillation with left bundle branch block (LBBB)

NOTE

- Recorded at half sensitivity (0.5 cm=1 mV)
- Irregular broad complex tachycardia
- No obvious P waves, but irregular baseline in lead VR
- LBBB configuration of QRS complexes

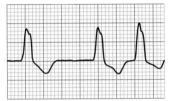

M wave of LBBB in lead V_6

The ECG in Fig. 4.26 shows a very irregular broad complex rhythm with no obvious P waves. There is an obvious LBBB pattern in leads V_5 and V_6. Whether the R–R interval is short or long, the appearance of the QRS complex is the same. The irregularity is the key to the diagnosis of atrial fibrillation with LBBB.

The ECG in Fig. 4.27 is also an example of atrial fibrillation and LBBB, but this is not quite as obvious as in Fig. 4.26. The QRS complexes at first sight may appear regular, but on close inspection they are not. The LBBB is also not so obvious, but can be seen in lead I.

Occasionally, it may be possible to identify P waves with a slower rate than the QRS complexes, indicating that the QRS complexes must be ventricular in origin. A 12-lead ECG during the tachycardia is important for this, because P waves may be visible in some leads but not in others (Fig. 4.28).

Atrial fibrillation with left bundle branch block (LBBB)

NOTE

- Broad complex rhythm at 140 bpm
- Slightly irregular rhythm, best seen in lead V_6
- LBBB pattern, most obvious in lead I

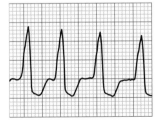

Irregular rhythm in lead V_6

Fig. 4.28

Ventricular tachycardia

P

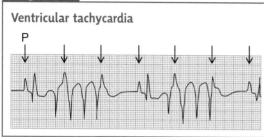

NOTE

- A single sinus beat is followed by a broad complex tachycardia
- During tachycardia, P waves can still be seen at a normal rate (arrowed)
- So the broad complex tachycardia must have a ventricular origin

Fig. 4.29

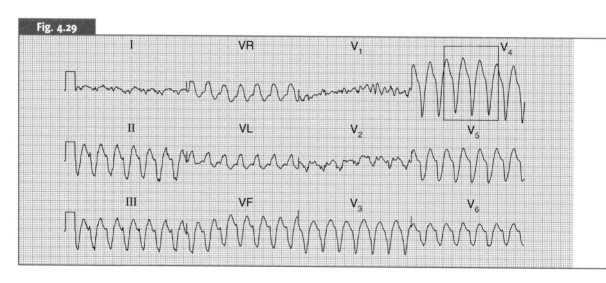

The QRS complex

The ECG in Fig. 4.29 shows a broad complex tachycardia recorded from a patient with an acute infarction, and there is no question that this represents VT.

The important features are:

- regular rhythm at 160 bpm (a fairly typical rate)
- very broad complexes of 360 ms duration (when the QRS complex duration is > 160 ms, VT is likely)
- left axis deviation
- in the V leads the QRS complexes all point in the same direction (in this case, downwards). This is called 'concordance'.

The ECG in Fig. 4.30 shows an ECG from another patient with an acute infarction. The shape of the QRS complexes is different from that in Fig. 4.29, but the principles are the same:

- The rhythm is regular.
- The complexes are very broad.
- There is left axis deviation.
- The complexes show concordance.

The ECG in Fig. 4.31 shows another example of VT, but this time the axis is normal. Unfortunately, the 'rules' for diagnosing VT are not absolute and one or more of the features above may not be present.

The ECG in Fig. 4.32 shows atrial fibrillation with an abnormal QRS complex, the duration of which (116 ms) is just within the normal range. The RSR^1 pattern, most obviously seen in lead V_2, and the slurred S wave in lead V_6, shows that this is partial RBBB. Note that the second R peak of the QRS complex (R^1) is higher than first peak. This is characteristic of RBBB. These features show that this is a supraventricular rhythm.

Ventricular tachycardia

NOTE

- Regular broad complex tachycardia, 160 bpm
- Appearance of lead V_1 is clearly an artefact
- Left axis deviation
- All complexes in the chest leads point downwards (concordance)
- There are no R waves in the chest leads, so the complexes are sometimes known as 'QS' complexes

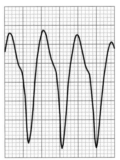

Broad complexes

Fig. 4.30

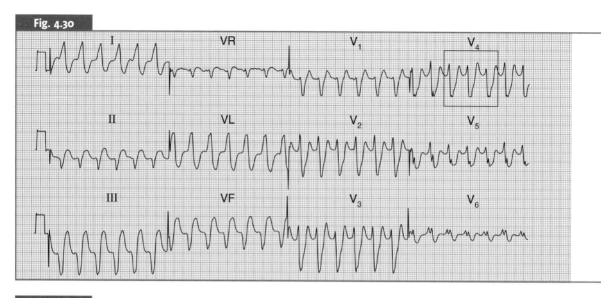

Fig. 4.31

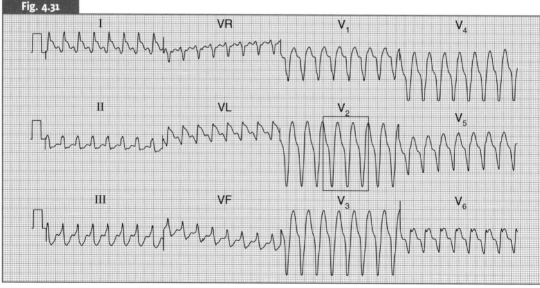

Ventricular tachycardia

NOTE

- Regular broad complex tachycardia, 150 bpm
- No P waves visible
- Left axis deviation
- Concordance (downward) of QRS complexes in the chest leads

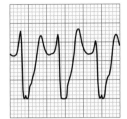

Broad complexes

Ventricular tachycardia

NOTE

- Regular broad complex tachycardia, 150 bpm
- No P waves visible
- Left axis deviation
- Concordance of QRS complexes in chest leads

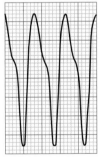

Broad complexes

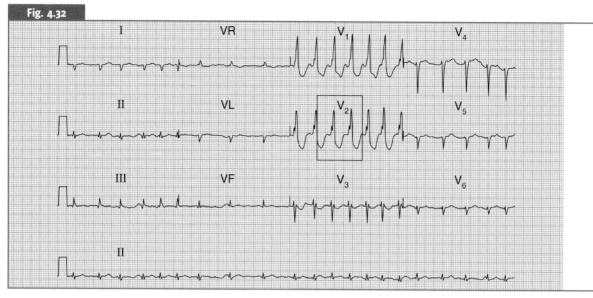

Fig. 4.32

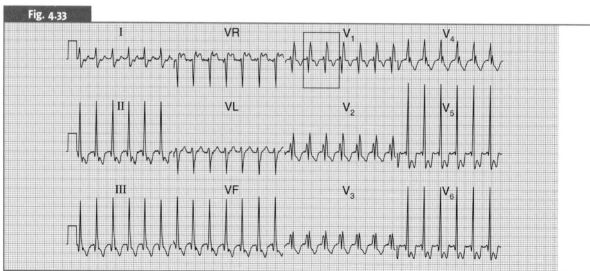

Fig. 4.33

Atrial fibrillation with right bundle branch block (RBBB)

NOTE

- Irregular broad complex tachycardia
- Right axis deviation
- QRS complexes show RBBB pattern, with second R peak higher than the first

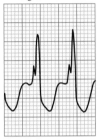

R^1 taller than R peak in lead V_2

Junctional tachycardia with right bundle branch block or ?fascicular tachycardia

NOTE

- Regular rhythm, 150 bpm
- Normal axis (R and S waves equal in lead I)
- QRS complex duration 120 ms (upper limit of normal)
- The second R peak (R^1) is taller than the R peak

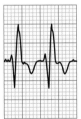

R^1 taller than R peak in lead V_1

The ECG in Fig. 4.33 shows a regular tachycardia with no P waves and a QRS complex showing an RBBB pattern. The duration of the QRS complex is at the upper limit of normal, at 120 ms. This might be a supraventricular tachycardia (probably AVNRT) with RBBB conduction, or it might be a fascicular tachycardia. A fascicular tachycardia usually arises in the posterior fascicle of the left bundle branch. Typically, there is left axis deviation (not present here). Fascicular tachycardia is an unusual rhythm with a benign prognosis, and it typically responds to verapamil.

The ECG in Fig. 4.34 shows how difficult differentiation between supraventricular and ventricular rhythms can be. Some features suggest a supraventricular, and some a ventricular, origin of the rhythm.

Often only a comparison of the patient's ECGs taken in sinus rhythm and when the tachycardia is present will establish the nature of the tachycardia. In the case of any patient with a tachycardia, it is essential to look through the old notes to see if any ECGs have been recorded previously. The ECG in Fig. 4.35 shows the broad complex tachycardia of a patient who was in pain and was hypotensive. He was cardioverted, and Fig. 4.36 shows the post-cardioversion record. The QRS complexes are narrow, so the arrhythmia must have been VT.

Fig. 4.34

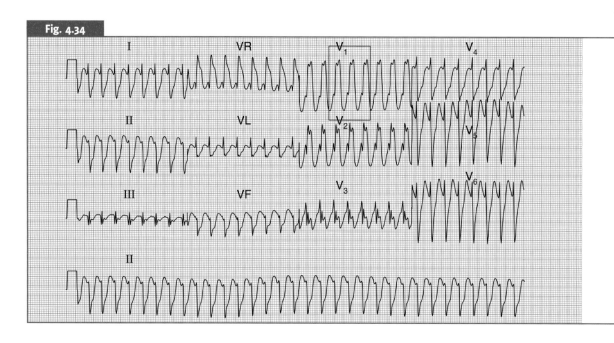

Fig. 4.35

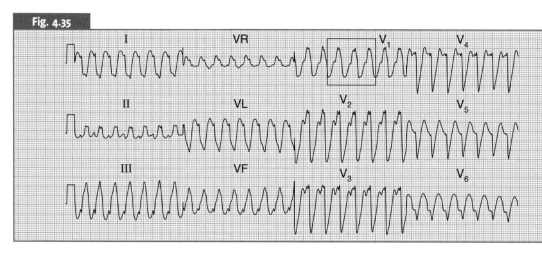

Broad complex tachycardia of uncertain origin

NOTE

- Regular rhythm, 195 bpm
- Right axis deviation (suggests a supraventricular tachycardia with bundle branch block)
- Very broad QRS complexes, with duration 200 ms (the primary evidence for ventricular tachycardia)
- QRS complexes in lead V_1 point upwards, while complexes in V_6 point downwards: no concordance (suggests a supraventricular tachycardia)
- The second R peak (R^1) is greater than the first R peak in lead V_1 (suggests a supraventricular tachycardia)

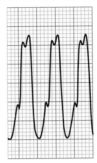

Broad complexes

Broad complex tachycardia: ?ventricular, ?supraventricular

NOTE

- Regular rhythm, 180 bpm
- Right axis deviation
- Very broad complexes, with QRS complex duration 200 ms
- R and R^1 peaks are variable
- No concordance

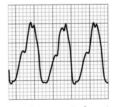

Variable R and R^1 peaks in lead V_1

Fig. 4.36

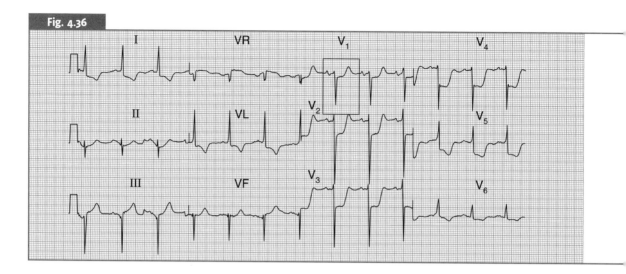

Fig. 4.37

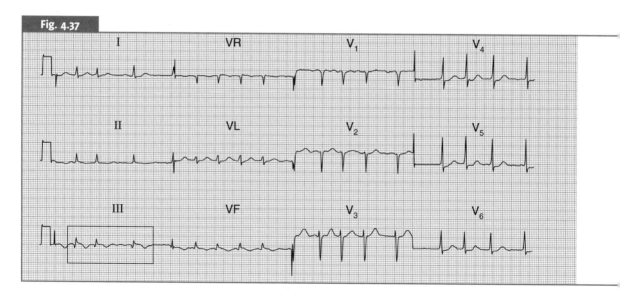

Post-cardioversion: sinus rhythm with normal conduction

NOTE

- Same patient as in Fig. 4.35
- Sinus rhythm
- Axis now shows left deviation
- Narrow QRS complexes
- Widespread ST segment depression, indicating ischaemia
- The narrow QRS complexes, with a change of axis, show that the original rhythm (shown in Fig. 4.35) must have been ventricular

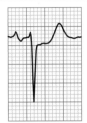

Narrow QRS complexes in lead V₁

Atrial fibrillation and inferior infarction

NOTE

- Irregular, narrow complex rhythm
- Irregular baseline indicates atrial fibrillation
- Normal axis
- Small Q waves in leads III and VF with inverted T waves, suggesting inferior infarction
- Slight ST segment depression in leads V_4–V_5 suggests ischaemia

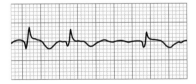

Small Q waves and inverted T waves in lead III

Fig. 4.37 shows the ECG from a patient admitted to a hospital with an inferior myocardial infarction, initially with atrial fibrillation. The patient then developed a broad complex tachycardia (Fig. 4.38). In the context of an acute infarction this would almost certainly be VT. A comparison of Figs 4.37 and 4.38 shows the development of a different, indeterminate, axis and of RBBB. The change of axis is a strong pointer to a ventricular origin of the rhythm.

Fusion beats and capture beats

If an early beat can be found with a narrow QRS complex, it can be assumed that a wide complex tachycardia is ventricular in origin. The narrow early beat demonstrates that the bundle branches will conduct supraventricular beats normally, even at high heart rates.

A 'fusion beat' is said to occur when the ventricles are activated simultaneously by a supraventricular and a ventricular impulse, so that a QRS complex with an intermediate pattern is seen (Fig. 4.39). The appearance of fusion beats is variable.

Fig. 4.38

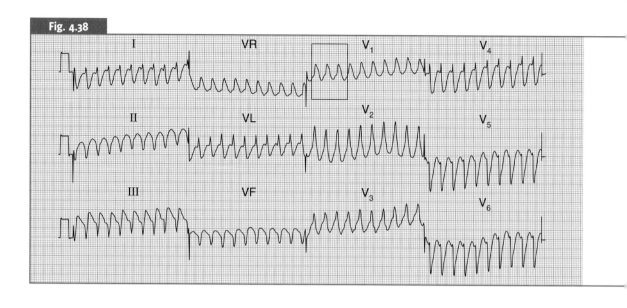

Fig. 4.39

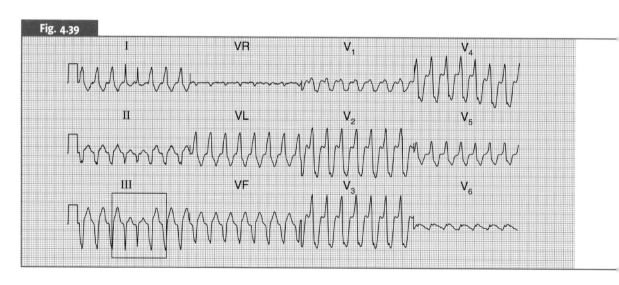

Ventricular tachycardia (VT) and inferior infarction

NOTE

- Same patient as in Fig. 4.37
- Broad complex tachycardia
- Indeterminate axis
- Right bundle branch block (RBBB) pattern, but in lead V_1, R peak greater than R^1 peak (not very clearly defined)
- No concordance
- With acute myocardial infarction, this will be VT

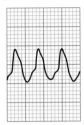

RBBB pattern in lead V_1

Ventricular tachycardia

NOTE

- Broad complex tachycardia, 180 bpm
- Left axis deviation
- Probable right bundle branch block (RBBB) pattern, with R peak greater than R^1 in lead V_1
- Two narrow complexes in leads I–III – the first is probably a 'fusion' beat and the second a 'capture' beat

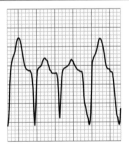

Fusion and capture beats in lead III

A 'capture beat' occurs when the ventricles are activated by an impulse of supraventricular origin during a run of VT (also shown in Fig. 4.39), and so capture beats have a QRS complex like those seen in a supraventricular rhythm. Fig. 4.40 shows another example of a capture beat, indicating that the broad complex tachycardia is VT.

Differentiation of broad complex tachycardias

Box 4.5 summarizes some distinguishing features of broad complex tachycardias.

Fig. 4.40

Ventricular tachycardia

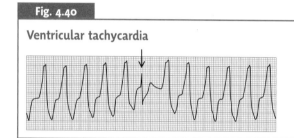

NOTE

- A single early beat with a narrow QRS complex (arrowed) interrupts a broad complex tachycardia
- A single 'capture' beat must have a supraventricular origin, and by inference the broad complexes must have a ventricular origin

---

Fig. 4.41

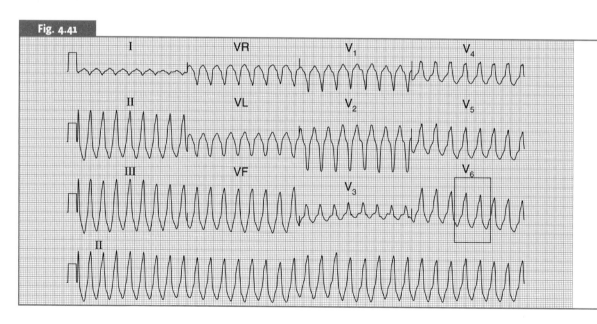

Special forms of VT in patients with symptoms
Right ventricular outflow tract ventricular tachycardia

This type of tachycardia, which originates in the right ventricular outflow tract, can be exercise-induced. It is recognizable because the broad complex tachycardia shows a combination of right axis deviation and LBBB (Fig. 4.41). RVOT-VT can be treated by ablation.

Torsade de pointes

VT is called 'monomorphic' when all QRS complexes have the same appearance, and 'polymorphic' when they vary. A 'twisting' or 'writhing' polymorphic VT is called 'torsade de pointes' (Fig. 4.42). This is often seen in patients whose ECG in sinus rhythm shows a long QT (Fig. 4.43; see Ch. 2, pp 72–75, and Ch. 8, Figs 8.20 and 8.21).

BOX 4.5 Differentiation of Broad Complex Tachycardias

- Broad complex tachycardias in patients with acute myocardial infarction are likely to be ventricular
- Compare with record taken in sinus rhythm–change of axis suggests a ventricular rhythm
- Left axis deviation, especially with right bundle branch block, is usually ventricular
- Identify P waves (independent P waves may be seen in ventricular tachycardia)
- QRS complex width: if > 160 ms, usually ventricular
- QRS complex regularity: if very irregular, probably atrial fibrillation with conduction defect
- Concordance: ventricular tachycardia is likely if the QRS complexes are predominantly upward, or predominantly downward, in all the chest leads
- With right bundle branch block pattern, ventricular origin is likely if:
  - there is left axis deviation
  - the primary R wave is taller than the secondary R wave (R^1) in lead V_1
- With left bundle branch block pattern, ventricular origin is likely if there is a QS wave (i.e. no R wave) in lead V_6
- Capture beats: narrow complex following short R–R interval (i.e. an early narrow beat interrupting a broad complex tachycardia) suggests that the basic rhythm is ventricular
- Fusion beats: an intermediate QRS complex pattern arises when the ventricles are activated simultaneously by a supraventricular and a ventricular impulse

---

Right ventricular outflow tract ventricular tachycardia
NOTE
- Broad complex tachycardia
- Right axis deviation
- Left bundle branch block (LBBB) pattern

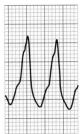

Broad QRS complexes and LBBB pattern in lead V_6

Fig. 4.42

Torsade de pointes ventricular tachycardia

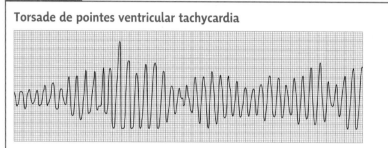

NOTE

- Broad complex, polymorphic tachycardia with continual change of shape

Fig. 4.43

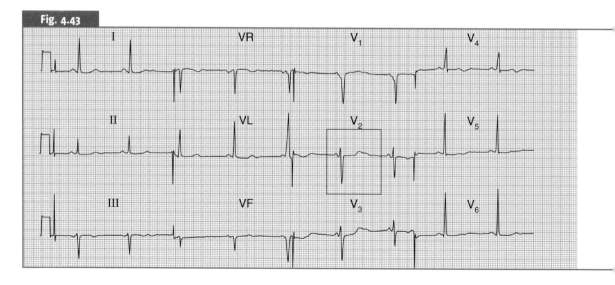

Broad complex tachycardia associated with the WPW syndrome

In patients with an accessory pathway due to the WPW syndrome, if conduction within the re-entry circuit is antidromic (see page 105), the ECG will show a wide QRS complex which can look remarkably like VT.

In a patient with the WPW syndrome and atrial fibrillation, the complexes will be polymorphic (variable-shape) and very irregular. This is extremely dangerous, because if the fast-conducting accessory pathway becomes involved and conducts depolarization associated with atrial flutter or fibrillation to the ventricles, the result can be ventricular fibrillation (Figs 4.44 and 4.45).

MANAGEMENT OF ARRHYTHMIAS

The acute and chronic medical management of each arrhythmia is beyond the scope of this book but readers are encouraged to refer to contemporary published guidelines for recommended treatment strategies.

Long QT syndrome: drug toxicity
NOTE
- Sinus rhythm
- Third complex in lead VL is probably a 'fusion' beat
- QT interval difficult to measure because of U waves, but probably about 540 ms

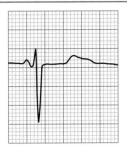

Long QT interval in lead V₂

Fig. 4.44

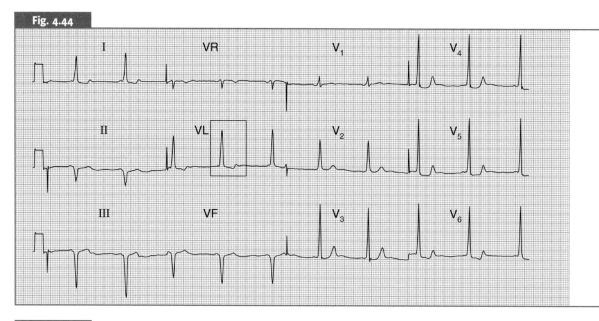

Fig. 4.45

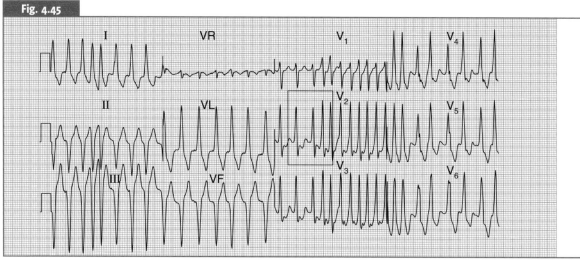

The Wolff–Parkinson–White syndrome, type A

NOTE

- Sinus rhythm
- Short PR interval
- Left axis deviation
- Prominent delta wave
- Dominant R waves in lead V_1, indicating type A WPW

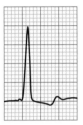

Short PR interval and delta wave in lead VL

ELECTROPHYSIOLOGY AND CATHETER ABLATION

The endocardial ECG

Electrical mapping catheters introduced via a transvenous route into the heart can be used to measure the pattern of electrical activation in the heart, the endocardial ECG. Usually, catheters are placed in the right atrium, the right ventricle, across the tricuspid valve (close to the His bundle) and in the coronary sinus (CS) to measure the pattern of left ventricular depolarization. Fig. 4.46 shows an X-ray taken during a fairly typical investigation, with exploring electrodes in different cardiac chambers. More sophisticated mapping catheters, including looped catheters and balloon catheters, may be employed in more complex cases.

Catheter ablation

If an abnormal conduction pathway, e.g. in the WPW syndrome, can be located (mapped) and permanently interrupted, a paroxysmal re-entry tachycardia can be

The Wolff–Parkinson–White syndrome with atrial fibrillation

NOTE

- Same patient as in Fig. 4.44
- Irregular broad complex tachycardia
- Rate up to 300 bpm
- Delta waves still apparent
- Marked irregularity suggests atrial fibrillation

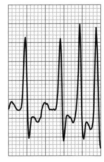

Delta waves in lead V_2

Fig. 4.46

Still fluoroscopic image of transvenous catheters during electrophysiology

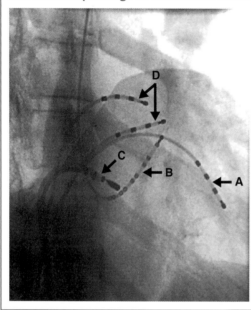

NOTE

- Catheters have multiple electrodes (dark bands) to enable mapping of the propagation of endocardial electrical activity
- Catheters shown are: right ventricular (A), coronary sinus (B), His bundle (C) and atrial (D)

prevented and the patient can be cured without the need for further drug therapy. This used to be done surgically, but now abnormal re-entry pathways are ablated (cauterized) by burning with radiofrequency energy applied through an intracardiac catheter. Ablation can also be used to destroy a focus of enhanced automaticity or triggered activity that is the cause of an arrhythmia.

The endocardial ECG is used to identify both the mechanism of an arrhythmia and the optimal position for the administration of a catheter-mediated radiofrequency ablation burn. The resting pattern of the cardiac electrical activity, as well as the pattern of activity in response

to atrial or ventricular pacing and attempted pharmacological stimulation of the arrhythmia, may be recorded during electrophysiological studies. Real-time analysis of the endocardial ECG allows the precise assessment of the relative timing of atrial and ventricular depolarization in different anatomical positions within the heart. This in turn provides information on the propagation of depolarization. Abnormal sources or routes of depolarization can then be mapped, and a position identified for radiofrequency ablation.

An example of the use of the endocardial ECG in catheter ablation is shown in Fig. 4.47. It is important to

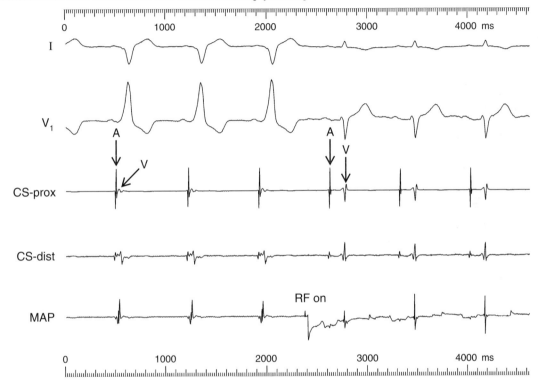

Fig. 4.47

Endocardial ECG: ablation of left-sided accessory pathway

NOTE
- Increased paper speed compared to 12-lead ECG
- Delta wave in first three beats: positive in lead V_1, negative in lead I, PR interval < 120 ms
- Atrial (A) and ventricular (V) depolarization are almost superimposed before ablation, indicating conduction via an accessory pathway
- After ablation (RF on): delta wave in leads I and V_1 is lost; increased PR interval (180 ms); increased separation of atrial and ventricular depolarization recorded in the coronary sinus. These changes indicate AV nodal conduction

recognize that the paper speed used in electrophysiology is usually greater than that used for 12-lead ECGs, and so the scale of the trace differs. Fig. 4.47 shows continuous traces from surface ECG leads I and V_1. Intracardiac electrograms are recorded at the proximal (CS-prox) and distal (CS-dist) poles of a multipolar catheter placed in the CS (Fig. 4.46). The CS runs in the groove of the left atrioventricular sulcus, so both atrial (A) and ventricular (V) electrograms are recorded. The atrial electrograms from the CS arise from atrial tissue close to the AV junction. These areas depolarize late in atrial systole, so they coincide with the end of the P wave seen in the surface ECG leads. The final electrogram shown in Fig. 4.47 was recorded from the tip of the mapping/ablation catheter (MAP). This single-tip catheter is used as a mapping electrode, to probe for the optimal site for ablation, and is also used to deliver the radiofrequency ablation burn once this position is found.

The first three beats recorded in Fig. 4.47 show sinus rhythm, conducted with pre-excitation via a left-sided accessory pathway – with a negative delta wave in lead I, positive delta wave in lead V_1; and closely spaced atrial (A) and ventricular (V) electrograms recorded by the CS catheter. On applying radiofrequency energy for ablation (RF on), there was an almost immediate loss of pre-excitation, with the disappearance of delta waves in the ECG leads in the following beats. The interval between atrial and ventricular electrograms within each beat increased at the CS catheter, indicating normal conduction via the AV node and no conduction via the accessory pathway. The PR interval also increased, from less than 120 ms in the first three beats to 180 ms, following successful radiofrequency ablation of the accessory pathway.

Arrhythmias amenable to ablation

Electrophysiology and catheter ablation is usually reserved for rhythms refractory to medical therapy. The following arrhythmias are potentially amenable to this approach.

Atrial flutter

Typical atrial flutter results from a re-entry circuit within the atria. This can be abolished by ablating an area known as the right atrial isthmus, which prevents re-entry from occurring (Fig. 4.48).

Atrial fibrillation

There is increasing evidence that, in a high proportion of patients, atrial fibrillation is initiated either by enhanced atrial automaticity or by triggered activity arising in the vicinity of the pulmonary veins, probably in atrial tissue extending into the pulmonary venous ostia and in the atrial area immediately outside the venous ostia. Ablation (Fig. 4.49) can isolate the atrial tissue within the pulmonary veins from the rest of the atrium, and hence can suppress the initiation of paroxysmal atrial fibrillation and also reduce relapse after the cardioversion of permanent atrial fibrillation.

The ablation treatment of atrial fibrillation is more difficult than that of atrial flutter, because the left atrium has to be entered through the inter-atrial septum, involving trans-septal puncture through the foramen ovale, and more burns are needed. It is usually initially performed with a wide-area circumferential ablation (WACA; denoted by red dots in Fig. 4.49). Further segmental ablation, guided by pacing from a CS electrode, may be required to eliminate persisting areas of conduction until the pulmonary veins are electrically silent. At present, this technique is usually regarded as a second-line option, limited to patients with symptoms refractory to conventional medical therapy, although its wider application is the subject of ongoing study.

AV node ablation

Patients with atrial-driven tachyarrhythmias, especially atrial fibrillation (whether paroxysmal or permanent), which cannot be controlled by pharmacological means, may undergo catheter ablation of the AV node. This leads

Fig. 4.48

Typical atrial flutter ablation

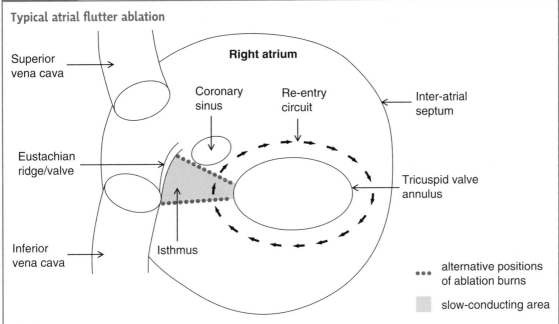

NOTE
- Arrhythmia occurs due to a clockwise or counter-clockwise re-entry circuit around the tricuspid valve annulus
- The re-entry circuit requires conduction through a narrow 'isthmus' of slow-conducting tissue (shaded grey) between the tricuspid valve annulus, the inferior vena cava, the coronary sinus and the Eustachian ridge/valve
- Radiofrequency ablation of this isthmus interrupts and prevents re-entry

Fig. 4.49

Ablation for atrial fibrillation

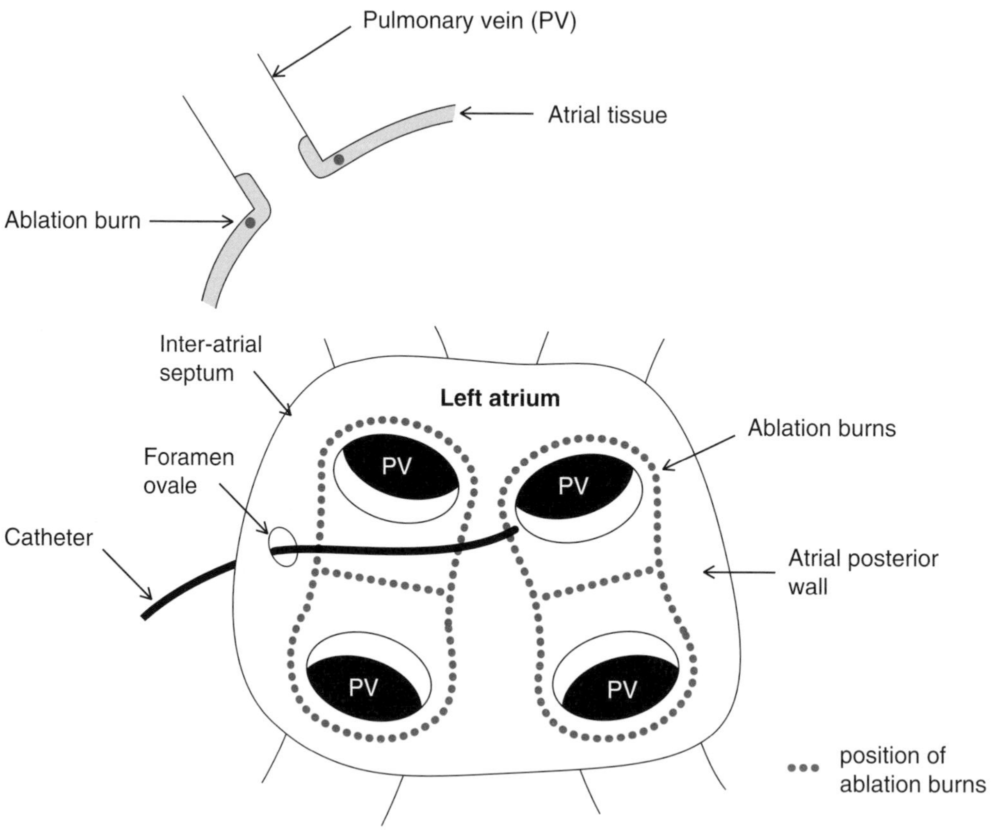

NOTE
- Anatomy of pulmonary venous drainage is variable. Most commonly four veins drain into the posterior left atrium

to complete AV block, and bradycardia is prevented by the implantation of a permanent pacemaker ('ablate and pace').

Pathway ablation

AVRTs, such as in the WPW syndrome, can be treated by ablation of the accessory pathway, as described above. This prevents re-entry and eliminates pre-excitation and episodes of supraventricular tachycardia. The ablation of pathways close to the AV node, including those involved in AVNRT, can be attempted. The aim of ablation is to modify the slow pathway, and so prevent AVNRT, without damaging the fast pathway, which would lead to AV block and necessitate a permanent pacemaker.

Ventricular tachycardia

Some forms of VT are amenable to catheter radiofrequency ablation treatment. These include RVOT-VT, where triggered activity is the cause, and also VT in some patients with surgically corrected congenital heart disease, if a simple ventricular re-entry circuit can be demonstrated. Ischaemic VT is a challenging substrate for electrophysiological ablation because often there are multiple potential foci of increased automaticity and potential re-entry circuits, due to areas of myocardial scarring. More sophisticated ventricular mapping tools are becoming available which potentially enable ablation treatment even for ischaemic VT.

Indications for electrophysiology

The indications for electrophysiology, and the associated hazards, are summarized in Box 4.6.

CARDIAC ARREST

The ECG in Fig. 4.50 was being recorded from a patient with an acute inferior myocardial infarction when he collapsed due to ventricular fibrillation (VF). Resuscitation should proceed according to current guidelines (see https://www.resus.org.uk/). Patients who survive ventricular fibrillation or VT with haemodynamic compromise outside the context of acute myocardial infarction should be considered for the insertion of an implanted cardioverter defibrillator (ICD) (see below).

ICD devices

These devices are designed for patients who have survived VF or are at increased risk of ventricular arrhythmia or sudden cardiac death. They have the following functions:
- pacemaker
- defibrillator
- control of VT.

Pacemaker function

ICD devices have the same functions as a conventional pacemaker (see Ch. 5). They can be single or dual chamber, or biventricular (cardiac resynchronisation therapy defibrillator; CRTD). In patients who do not require the pacing function, the ICD will usually be a single-chamber system, programmed as a backup VVI. The device will then be in continuous sensing mode.

Defibrillator function

The chest X-ray appearances of ICD devices are similar to those of conventional pacemakers. However, devices with a defibrillating function are bigger, incorporating more battery power for the delivery of shocks. In addition, the right ventricular lead contains the two poles of the shocking coil and so is thicker than a conventional lead (Fig. 4.51). Extracardiac devices are also available in which the shocking coil and defibrillator box act as electrodes and are placed subcutaneously in an arc around the chest wall rather than transvenously (Fig. 4.52).

In addition to the normal sensing functions of a pacemaker, an ICD can sense high rates of ventricular activity. If a predetermined ventricular rate is exceeded, an electrical shock discharges between the two poles of the

BOX 4.6 Indications and Complications of Electrophysiology

Indications

- Atrioventricular re-entry tachycardias, including the Wolff–Parkinson–White syndrome
- Atrial fibrillation or atrial flutter, either paroxysmal or permanent, where the symptoms are refractory to conventional therapy or where medical therapy is contraindicated or poorly tolerated
- AV node ablation for paroxysmal or permanent atrial arrhythmias (especially atrial fibrillation) refractory to rate control with conventional medical therapy
- AV node slow pathway modification for symptomatic/medication-refractory AVNRT
- Ventricular tachycardias including those associated with congenital heart disease and right ventricular outflow tract ventricular tachycardia
- Symptomatic or frequent ventricular extrasystoles, especially if associated with a significant cardiomyopathy

Complications

- Peri-procedural stroke or transient ischaemic attack (TIA) (1%)
- Groin haematoma (7%)
- Pericardial tamponade (1%)
- Arteriovenous fistula (< 1%)
- Higher degree AV block (with pathways close to the AV node)
- Pulmonary vein stenosis (1%) (pulmonary vein isolation only)
- Repeated procedures (complex studies may require repeat procedures)

Fig. 4.50

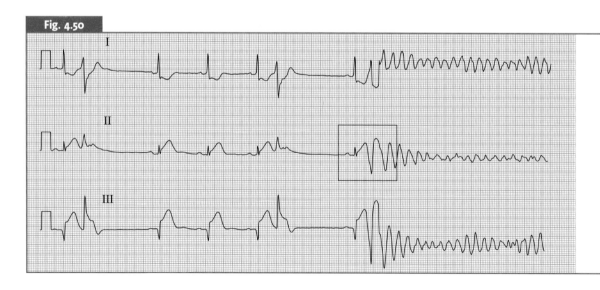

defibrillator coil in the ventricular lead (or between the defibrillator coil and the device can), with the aim of cardioverting a life-threatening ventricular arrhythmia (Fig. 4.53). If the ventricular rate does not fall below the threshold following one shock, then further shocks may be delivered.

Anti-tachycardia pacing

The device may also attempt to control VT by 'overdrive pacing'. If ventricular activity is detected within a certain range (usually significantly above normal cardiac rates but below the threshold set for defibrillation), the ICD will attempt to pace the ventricle at a high rate before reducing the rate of pacing. Ventricular capture with rapid pacing can sometimes terminate VT. New extra-cardiac defibrillator devices are being developed which can communicate wirelessly with an implanted leadless pacemaker to enable anti-tachycardia pacing in a fully leadless combined device. If anti-tachycardia pacing in this way is unsuccessful after a set number of attempts, the ICD will usually default to defibrillation.

Indications for ICD devices

These are summarized in Box 4.7.

ECG appearance

ECGs from patients with ICDs are the same as those from patients with conventional pacemakers, except when a ventricular arrhythmia is detected.

Abnormal ICD function

Either the pacing function or the defibrillator function of an ICD device may rarely fail. The defibrillator

---

Ventricular fibrillation

NOTE

- Leads I, II and III, continuous records
- Initially sinus rhythm, with occasional ventricular extrasystoles
- R on T ventricular extrasystole followed by ventricular fibrillation

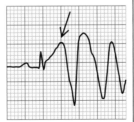

R on T phenomenon in lead II

BOX 4.7 Indications for ICD Insertion

'Primary' prevention

- Heart failure and ejection fraction < 35% and QRS complexes > 120 ms
- Heart failure and ejection fraction < 35% and QRS complexes < 120 ms if at high risk of sudden cardiac death
- Familial risk of sudden cardiac death including hypertrophic cardiomyopathy, long QT syndrome, Brugada syndrome, or ARVD (arrhythmogenic right ventricular dysplasia)
- Surgical repair of congenital heart disease

Secondary prevention

- Survived cardiac arrest due to ventricular fibrillation or VT
- Spontaneous sustained VT causing syncope or haemodynamic compromise
- Sustained VT and ejection fraction < 35% (but symptoms no worse that NYHA Class III)

Note: CRT with ICD (CRT-D) is indicated for primary prevention in situations where the QRS duration in more prolonged.

Fig. 4.51

Single chamber ICD

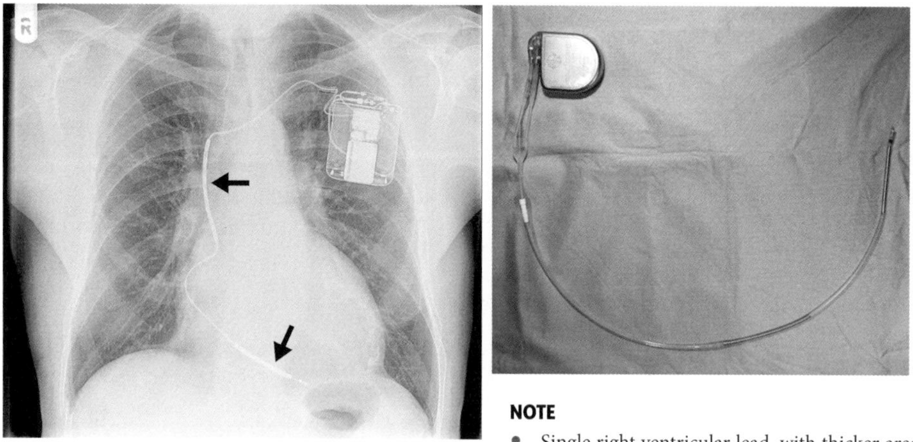

NOTE
- Single right ventricular lead, with thicker areas indicating the poles of the shocking coils (arrowed)

function may either fail appropriately to initiate ventricular arrhythmia therapy, or may deliver inappropriate shocks. This will require specialist input and analysis. In the event of inappropriate repeated shock delivery, an ICD can be inactivated in a monitored patient by the application of a magnet.

ICDs should always be interrogated shortly after shock delivery, even if this was appropriate, to check device function and battery life. The presence of pacemakers or ICDs in no way precludes external defibrillation, provided that the paddles are not applied directly over the device.

Fig. 4.52

Subcutaneous ICD

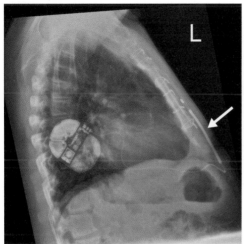

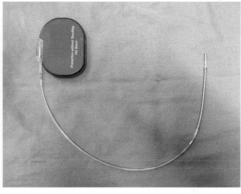

NOTE
- Lead runs subcutaneously such that the shocking coils (arrowed) run close to the sternum
- The other pole for defibrillation is provided by the device can

Fig. 4.53

ICD cardioversion of ventricular fibrillation

NOTE
- Ventricular fibrillation (1) followed by ICD-mediated cardioversion (2)
- Intrinsic QRS complexes (3)
- Paced ventricular responses (4)

The ECG when the patient has a bradycardia $\Large 5$

Mechanism of bradycardias	**147**
Sinoatrial disease – the 'sick sinus syndrome'	147
Atrial fibrillation and flutter	154
AV block	157
Management of bradycardias	**163**
Temporary pacing in patients with acute myocardial infarction	163
Permanent pacing	163
Right ventricular pacemakers (VVI)	170
Right atrial pacemakers (AAI)	183
Dual-chamber pacemakers (DDD)	185
Abnormal pacemaker function	188
Indications for pacemaker insertion	191

MECHANISM OF BRADYCARDIAS

Patients are seldom aware that their heart rate is slow, but they can certainly be aware of the effects of a bradycardia. Marked sinus bradycardia is characteristic of athletic training but bradycardia is also a contributory cause of: the symptom of fainting in vasovagal attacks; the reduced cardiac output and syncope associated with heart block; and the hypotension and heart failure in patients with an inferior myocardial infarction. A slow heart rate can also be a major contributor to angina. An ECG is therefore an essential part of the investigation of any patient with a slow pulse rate, and indeed of any patient with dizziness, syncope or breathlessness.

The causes of sinus bradycardia have been discussed in Chapter 1 (see p. 5 and Box 1.2, p. 7). Escape rhythms have been discussed in Chapter 2 (p. 77). They are usually asymptomatic, but symptoms occur when the automaticity that generates the escape rhythm is inadequate to maintain a cardiac output. A bradycardia may cause the symptom of syncope; some of the possible underlying causes are listed in Box 5.1.

Sinoatrial disease – the 'sick sinus syndrome'

Disordered sinoatrial (SA) node function can be familial or congenital and can occur in ischaemic, valvular, hypertensive or infiltrative cardiac disease. It is, however, frequently idiopathic. Abnormal function of the SA node may be associated with failure of the conduction system. Patients with SA disease may be asymptomatic, but all the symptoms associated with bradycardias – dizziness,

BOX 5.1 Conditions Associated With Syncope

Atrial fibrillation with slow ventricular rate
- Valvular heart disease
- Ischaemic heart disease
- Cardiomyopathies
- Drugs:
  - digoxin
  - beta-blockers
  - verapamil
  - amiodarone

'Sick sinus' disease
- Congenital
- Familial
- Idiopathic
- Ischaemic heart disease
- Cardiomyopathy

- Amyloidosis
- Collagen diseases
- Myocarditis
- Drugs, e.g. lithium

Second or third degree block
- Idiopathic (fibrosis)
- Congenital
- Ischaemia
- Aortic valve calcification
- Surgery or trauma
- Tumours in the His bundle
- Drugs:
  - digoxin
  - beta-blockers
  - verapamil

Fig. 5.1

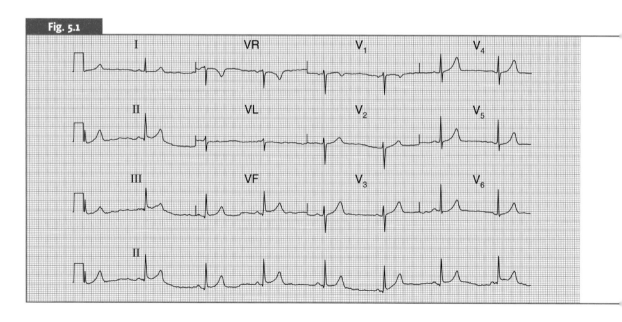

syncope and the symptoms of heart failure – can occur. Atrial and junctional tachycardias often occur together with sinus node dysfunction, when the patient may present with palpitations.

The abnormal rhythms seen in the sick sinus syndrome are listed in Box 5.2.

The ECGs in Figs 5.1 and 5.2 are from a young man who had a normal ECG with a slow sinus rate when asymptomatic, but intermittently became extremely dizzy when he developed a profound sinus bradycardia.

The ECG in Fig. 5.3 shows an ambulatory record from a young woman who complained of short-lived attacks of dizziness. When she had these, the ECG showed sinus pauses.

BOX 5.2 Cardiac Rhythms in the Sick Sinus Syndrome

- Unexplained or inappropriate sinus bradycardia
- Sudden changes in sinus rate
- Sinus pauses (sinoatrial arrest or exit block)
- Atrial standstill ('silent atrium')
- Atrioventricular junctional escape rhythms
- Atrial tachycardia alternating with junctional escape (bradycardia–tachycardia syndrome)
- Junctional tachycardia alternating with junctional escape
- Atrial fibrillation with a slow ventricular response

Sinus bradycardia
NOTE
- Sinus rhythm
- Rate 45 bpm, ECG otherwise normal

Fig. 5.2

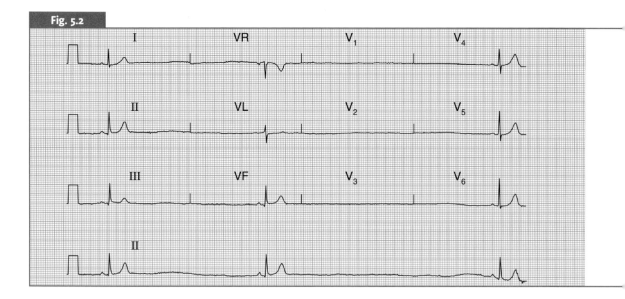

Fig. 5.3

Sinus pauses

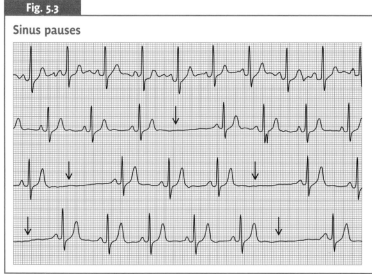

NOTE

- Ambulatory record
- Sinus rhythm throughout, but marked pauses (arrowed) at time of symptoms
- In the pause, the P–P interval is exactly twice the P–P interval of the preceding beat. There has therefore been 'exit block' from the SA node

Fig. 5.4 shows the other variety of sinus pause – sinus arrest.

The ECG in Fig. 5.5 shows an example of a 'silent atrium', when the heart rhythm depends on the irregular depolarization of a focus in the atrioventricular (AV) node.

The combination of sick sinus syndrome and episodes of tachycardia is sometimes called the 'tachycardia–bradycardia syndrome', and Fig. 5.6 shows the rhythm of a patient with this syndrome. This patient was asymptomatic at times, when his ECG showed a 'silent atrium' with a slow and irregular junctional (AV nodal) escape rhythm, but he complained of palpitations when he had an AV nodal tachycardia.

Sick sinus syndrome: sinus bradycardia

NOTE

- Same patient as in Fig. 5.1
- Sinus rhythm
- Rate down to 12 bpm at times
- No complexes recorded in leads V_1–V_3

Fig. 5.4

Sinus arrest

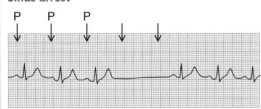

NOTE

- Sinus rhythm
- After three beats, there is a 'sinus pause' with no P wave
- Arrows mark where the next two P waves should have been
- Sinus rhythm is then restored, but the cycle has been reset

Fig. 5.5

Sick sinus syndrome: silent atrium

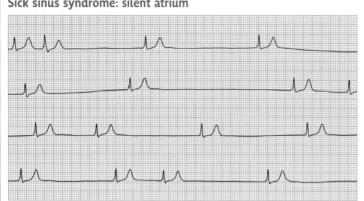

NOTE
- Ambulatory recording from lead II
- Irregular, narrow complex rhythm
- No P waves visible
- Nodal escape, with rate down to 16 bpm at times

Fig. 5.7

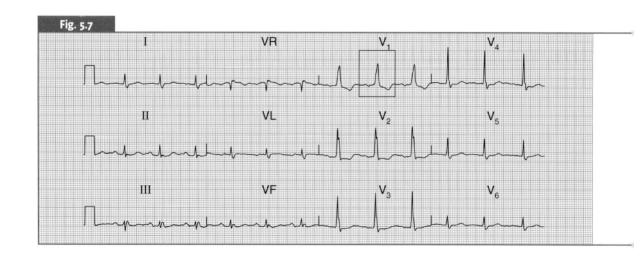

Fig. 5.6

Sick sinus syndrome: bradycardia–tachycardia syndrome

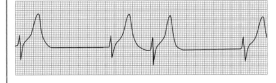

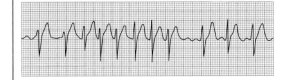

NOTE

- Upper trace: a silent atrium with irregular junctional escape beats
- Lower trace: junctional tachycardia is followed by a period of sinus rhythm

First degree block and right bundle branch block
NOTE

- Sinus rhythm
- PR interval 220 ms (first degree block)
- Right bundle branch block (RBBB)

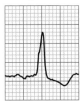

Long PR interval and RBBB pattern in lead V$_1$

Fig. 5.7 shows the ECG from a patient who, when asymptomatic, showed first degree block and right bundle branch block suggesting a potential for higher degree AV block. He complained of fainting attacks, but an ambulatory recording showed that this in fact due to sinus arrest with a very slow AV nodal escape rhythm, giving a ventricular rate of 15 bpm (Fig. 5.8). This is an example of the combination of conduction system disease and sick sinus syndrome.

Possible causes of sick sinus syndrome are listed in Box 5.3.

Fig. 5.8

Sinus arrest and atrioventricular nodal escape

NOTE

- Same patient as in Fig. 5.7
- Ambulatory record
- No P waves
- Narrow complex rhythm
- Rate 15 bpm, due to AV nodal (junctional) escape

Atrial fibrillation and flutter

A slow ventricular rate can accompany atrial flutter or atrial fibrillation because of slow conduction through the AV node and His bundle systems (Figs 5.9 and 5.10). This may be the result of treatment with drugs that delay AV nodal conduction, such as digoxin, beta-blockers or verapamil, but can occur because of conducting tissue disease.

Complete block associated with atrial fibrillation is recognized from the regular and wide QRS complexes which originate in the ventricular muscle (Fig. 5.11).

Fig. 5.9

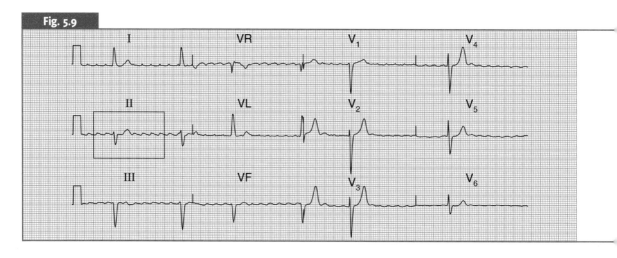

BOX 5.3 Causes of the Sick Sinus Syndrome

Familial
- Isolated
- With atrioventricular conduction disturbance
- With QT interval prolongation
- Congenital

Acquired
- Idiopathic
- Coronary disease
- Valvular heart disease
- Cardiomyopathy
- Neuromuscular disease:
  - Friedreich's ataxia
  - peroneal muscular atrophy
  - Charcot–Marie–Tooth disease

- Infiltration:
  - amyloidosis
  - haemochromatosis
- Collagen diseases:
  - rheumatoid
  - scleroderma
  - systemic lupus erythematosus
- Myocarditis:
  - viral
  - diphtheria
- Drugs:
  - lithium
  - Ivabradine
  - aerosol propellants

Atrial flutter with variable block
NOTE
- Irregular bradycardia
- Flutter waves at 300 bpm obvious in all leads
- Ventricular rate varies, range 30–55 bpm
- QRS complex duration slightly prolonged (128 ms), indicating partial right bundle branch block
- There is not complete block, as shown by the irregular QRS complexes

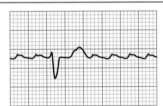

Flutter waves in lead II

Fig. 5.10

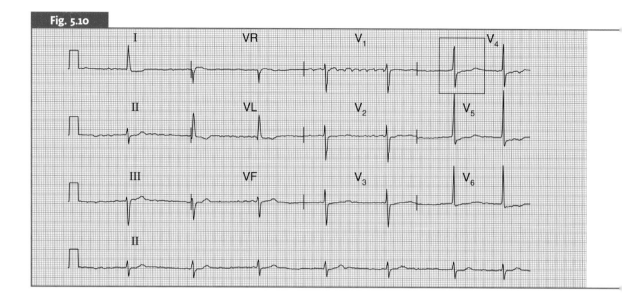

Fig. 5.11

Atrial fibrillation and complete block

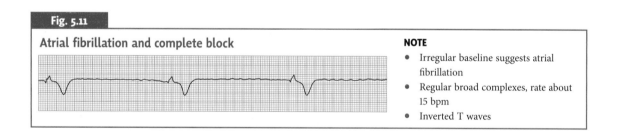

NOTE
- Irregular baseline suggests atrial fibrillation
- Regular broad complexes, rate about 15 bpm
- Inverted T waves

Atrial fibrillation

NOTE

- Irregular rhythm, rate 43 bpm
- Flutter-like waves in lead V_1 but these are not constant
- Left axis deviation
- QRS complexes otherwise normal
- Prolonged QT intervals of 530 ms: ?hypokalaemia

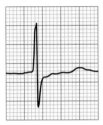

Prolonged QT interval in lead V_4

AV block

Symptoms are not caused by first degree block, second degree block of the Wenckebach or Mobitz type 2 varieties, left anterior hemiblock or the bundle branch blocks.

Second degree block of the 2:1 or 3:1 type will cause dizziness and breathlessness if the ventricular rate is slow enough (Fig. 5.12). Young people tolerate slow hearts better than old people do.

Complete (third degree) block characteristically involves a slow rate, but this may be fast enough to cause only tiredness or the symptoms of heart failure. Fig. 5.13 shows the ECG of a 60-year-old man who, despite a heart rate of 40 bpm, had few complaints.

If the ventricular rate is very slow the patient may lose consciousness in a 'Stokes–Adams' attack, which can cause a seizure and sometimes death. The ECG in Fig. 5.14 is from a patient who was asymptomatic while his ECG

Fig. 5.12

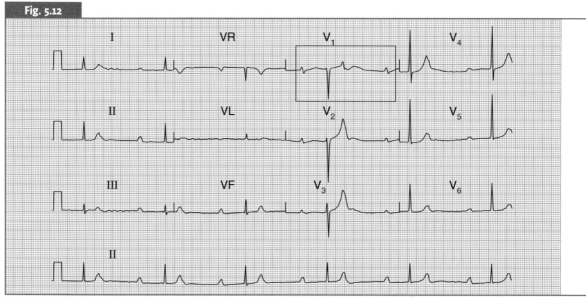

Fig. 5.13

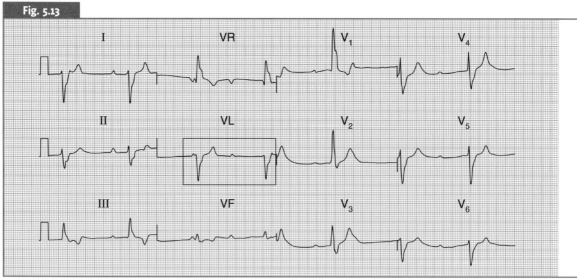

Second degree block (2:1)

NOTE

- Sinus rhythm
- Second degree block, 2:1 type
- Ventricular rate 33 bpm
- Long PR interval in the conducted beats (not characteristic of second degree block)
- Normal QRS complexes and T waves

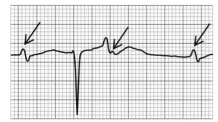

P waves in lead V₁

Complete heart block

NOTE

- Sinus rate 70 bpm
- Regular ventricular rate, 40 bpm
- No relationship between P waves and QRS complexes
- Wide QRS complexes
- Right bundle branch block pattern

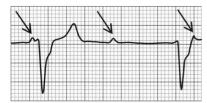

P waves in lead VL

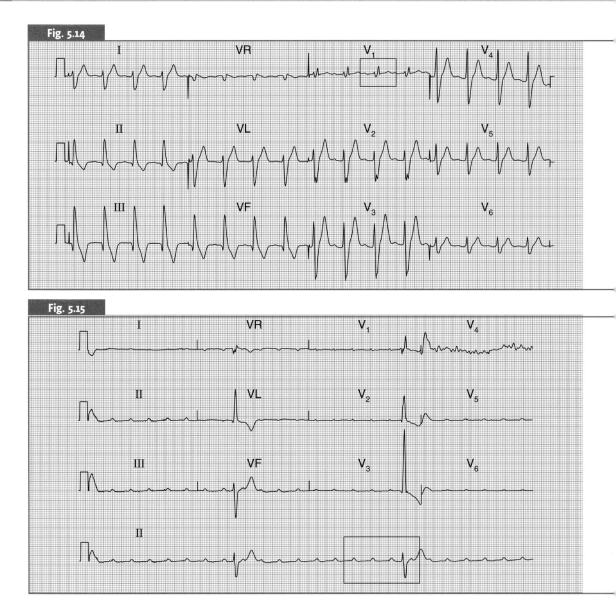

Fig. 5.14

Fig. 5.15

First degree block and right bundle branch block

NOTE

- Sinus rhythm
- PR interval 240 ms
- Right axis deviation
- Right bundle branch block (RBBB)

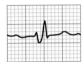

Long PR interval and RBBB pattern in lead V₁

Complete block and Stokes–Adams attack

NOTE

- Same patient as in Fig. 5.14
- Sinus rate 140 bpm
- Ventricular rate 15 bpm
- No relationship between P waves and QRS complexes
- Because of the slow ventricular rate, no QRS complexes were recorded in leads I–III or V₄–V₆, although the rhythm strip shows a complex in lead II

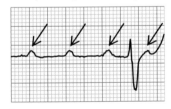

P waves

showed sinus rhythm with first degree block and right bundle branch block, but who then had a Stokes–Adams attack with the onset of complete block (Fig. 5.15).

The possible causes of heart block are summarized in Box 5.4.

The endocardial ECG in AV block

The ordinary surface ECG provides all the information necessary for the identification of heart block, but the spread of excitation through the heart can be seen more accurately from an intracardiac recording.

The endocardial ECG used during electrophysiological studies simultaneously displays depolarizations recorded from several catheters, passed percutaneously via a vein in to the heart. Each catheter has multiple electrodes (see Fig. 4.46), which show the timing of depolarization through the heart (Fig. 5.16). The components of the wave of depolarization are best illustrated from recordings taken by the His catheter. The 'A' wave of atrial

BOX 5.4 Causes of Heart Block

First and second degree block
- Normal variant
- Increased vagal tone
- Athletes
- Sick sinus syndrome
- Acute carditis
- Ischaemic disease
- Hypokalaemia
- Lyme disease (*Borrelia burgdorferi*)
- Digoxin
- Beta-blockers
- Calcium-channel blockers

Complete block
- Idiopathic (conduction tissue fibrosis)
- Congenital
- Ischaemic disease
- Associated with aortic valve calcification
- Cardiac surgery and trauma
- Digoxin intoxication
- Bundle interruption by tumours, parasites, abscesses, granulomas, injury

Fig. 5.16

Normal His bundle electrogram

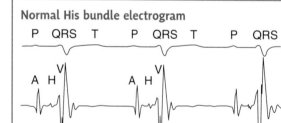

NOTE
- Upper trace shows the usual ECG recorded from the body surface
- The P waves, QRS complexes and T waves are broad and flat because the record made with a faster paper speed than normal
- The lower trace shows the intracardiac recording. The A and V waves correspond to the P waves and QRS complexes, but have a totally different appearance
- His bundle depolarization is shown as small spike labelled 'H'

Fig. 5.17

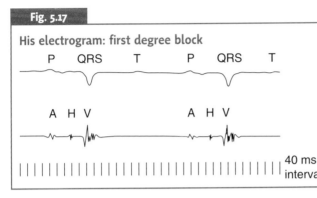

His electrogram: first degree block

NOTE
- Upper record shows surface ECG
- PR interval 200 ms
- Lower record shows His electrogram
- AH interval is prolonged (150 ms), but the HV interval is normal (70 ms)

depolarization (the P wave of the surface ECG) is normally followed by the sharp deflection of the 'H' spike, caused by the depolarization of the His bundle. The AH interval is 55–120 ms in normal subjects, with most of this period being due to delay within the AV node. The 'V' wave normally follows, representing ventricular depolarization (the QRS complex of the surface ECG). The HV interval (normal range 33–35 ms) measures the time taken for depolarization to spread from the His bundle to the first part of the interventricular septum.

Fig. 5.17 shows an endocardial ECG from a patient with first degree heart block, in this case due to prolongation of the AH interval.

A His bundle electrogram also demonstrates the site of second degree block. In the case of 2:1 block, this is usually in the His bundle rather than the AV node. Therefore, a normal H (or His) spike will be seen, but in the non-conducted beats the H spike will not be followed by a V wave (Figs 5.18 and 5.19).

MANAGEMENT OF BRADYCARDIAS

Bradycardias must be treated if they are associated with hypotension, poor peripheral perfusion, or escape arrhythmias.

Temporary pacing in patients with acute myocardial infarction

Bradyarrhythmias associated with an acute myocardial infarction, especially those with an inferior infarction, usually resolve spontaneously without the need for pacemaker insertion. Occasionally temporary pacing is required where bradycardia is profound or leads to syncope or heart failure.

Permanent pacing

Pacemakers and other cardiac devices are increasingly prevalent, especially in elderly patients. Although usually implanted and monitored by specialists, these devices are frequently encountered in a broad range of clinical contexts. The different types of pacemakers can be characterized by the number of cardiac chambers involved. Patients often carry a card indicating the type of device implanted, but this can also be determined by its characteristic appearance on a plain chest X-ray. A chest X-ray is, therefore, a useful part of any pacemaker assessment, and so this chapter includes a series of X-rays. It is essential that the type of device be determined before the ECG can be interpreted.

All pacemakers perform two fundamental functions: pacing and sensing. Most ECG findings in both normal

Fig. 5.18

Second degree block (2:1)

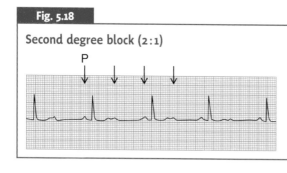

NOTE

- The conducted beats have a normal PR interval
- Alternate P waves are not followed by a QRS complex

Fig. 5.19

His electrogram: second degree block

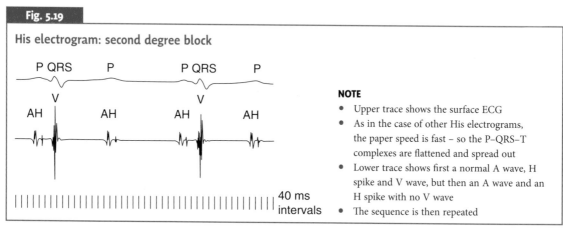

40 ms intervals

NOTE

- Upper trace shows the surface ECG
- As in the case of other His electrograms, the paper speed is fast – so the P–QRS–T complexes are flattened and spread out
- Lower trace shows first a normal A wave, H spike and V wave, but then an A wave and an H spike with no V wave
- The sequence is then repeated

and abnormal pacemaker functions can be explained in terms of pacing and sensing functions.

Pacing

An electrical pulse is generated between an electrical pole at the tip of the pacing lead and either a second pole more proximally within the pacing lead (bipolar lead) or the pacemaker box itself (unipolar lead). This causes depolarization of the surrounding myocardium, the propagation of an action potential from this focus and the contraction of the paced cardiac chamber. This process is repeated at a basal rate determined when the pacemaker is programmed, although it can be suppressed as a result of device sensing (see below).

Sensing

The pacemaker continuously monitors electrical activity in the vicinity of the tip of the pacing lead.

If intrinsic cardiac depolarization is sensed in a single-chamber pacemaker, the pacemaker will inhibit

Fig. 5.20

Pacemaker interrogation

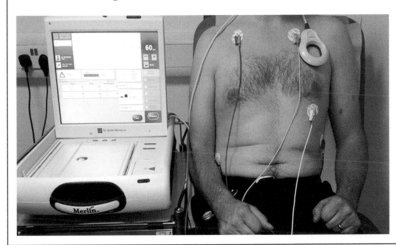

A header is placed over the pacemaker device (left shoulder) and ECG leads connected to the device programmer (screen to patient's right). The device can then be interrogated and programmed as required.

pacing for a predetermined period. This prevents simultaneous pacing in the presence of spontaneous cardiac activity.

In dual-chamber pacemakers, sensing depolarization can either inhibit pacing in the same chamber or trigger pacing in a different chamber. For example, if an intrinsic ventricular beat is sensed, ventricular pacing will be inhibited for a period. If atrial depolarization is sensed, ventricular pacing will be triggered after a programmed PR interval, but only if no ventricular activity has been sensed. Thus ventricular pacing can track atrial activity in the presence of AV block, leading to appropriate coordination of atrial and ventricular systoles.

Monitoring

Many modern pacemakers also have telemetry functions which, if enabled, can allow some ECG monitoring functions (similar to implantable loop recorders). Traditionally,

pacemakers were interrogated by application of a header to the skin over the device (Fig. 5.20). A device-specific analyser was then required to upload and print key pacing parameters (Figs 5.21 and 5.22). These include basic measures of battery life, and parameters to assess lead function but also details of how the device is working (such as the proportion of paced and sensed beats). Modern devices often allow home monitoring where the device connects wirelessly to a hub which can then relay these parameters to the hospital without requiring a patient visit.

Pacemaker nomenclature

The pacing mode of most pacemaker systems can be described using the NBG Code (NASPE/BPEG Generic, developed by the North American Society of Pacing and Electrophysiology Mode Code Committee and the British Pacing and Electrophysiology Group).

Fig. 5.21

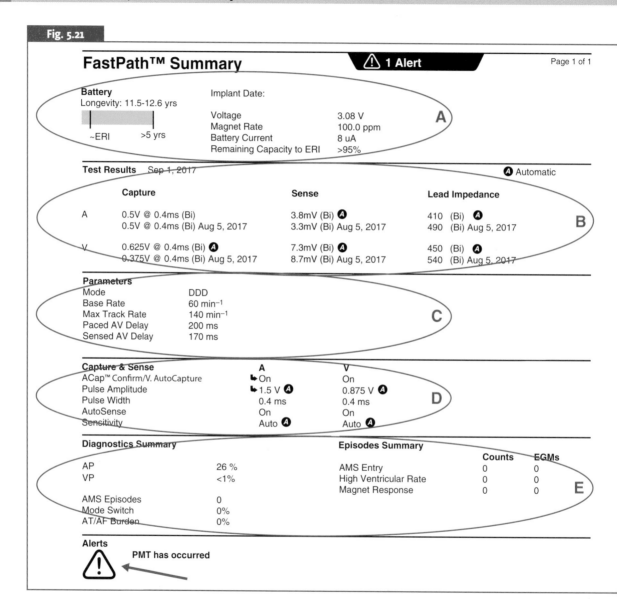

FastPath™ Summary ⚠ 1 Alert   Page 1 of 1

Battery
Longevity: 11.5-12.6 yrs

Implant Date:

~ERI   >5 yrs

Voltage	3.08 V
Magnet Rate	100.0 ppm
Battery Current	8 uA
Remaining Capacity to ERI	>95%

A

Test Results   Sep 1, 2017   **Ⓐ** Automatic

	Capture	Sense	Lead Impedance
A	0.5V @ 0.4ms (Bi)	3.8mV (Bi) Ⓐ	410 (Bi) Ⓐ
	0.5V @ 0.4ms (Bi) Aug 5, 2017	3.3mV (Bi) Aug 5, 2017	490 (Bi) Aug 5, 2017
V	0.625V @ 0.4ms (Bi) Ⓐ	7.3mV (Bi) Ⓐ	450 (Bi) Ⓐ
	0.375V @ 0.4ms (Bi) Aug 5, 2017	8.7mV (Bi) Aug 5, 2017	540 (Bi) Aug 5, 2017

B

Parameters

Mode	DDD
Base Rate	60 min⁻¹
Max Track Rate	140 min⁻¹
Paced AV Delay	200 ms
Sensed AV Delay	170 ms

C

Capture & Sense

	A	V
ACap™ Confirm/V. AutoCapture	↳On	On
Pulse Amplitude	↳1.5 V Ⓐ	0.875 V Ⓐ
Pulse Width	0.4 ms	0.4 ms
AutoSense	On	On
Sensitivity	Auto Ⓐ	Auto Ⓐ

D

Diagnostics Summary

		Episodes Summary	Counts	EGMs
AP	26 %	AMS Entry	0	0
VP	<1%	High Ventricular Rate	0	0
		Magnet Response	0	0
AMS Episodes	0			
Mode Switch	0%			
AT/AF Burden	0%			

E

Alerts

⚠ PMT has occurred

166

Pacemaker interrogation summary. (A) Battery life;
(B) lead parameters; (C and D) the current pacemaker
programming; (E) diagnostics. AP is the percentage of
atrial beats paced and VP is the percentage of ventricular
beats paced

Fig. 5.22

Heart Rate Histogram   Since Aug 5, 2017

Atrial

AF Suppression™   n/a

- ■ Paced (AP)
- □ Sensed (AS)
- ○ Sensor-Indicated Rate

Ventricular

Time at Max Track Rate   <1%
PMT Detections   1

- ■ Paced (AS-VP, AP-VP)
- □ Sensed (AS-VS, AP-VS)
- ■ PVC
- ○ Sensor-Indicated Rate

Excludes time in AMS

1: III AutoGain (31.0 mm/mV)
2: Markers
3: A Unipolar Ring AutoGain (4.6 mm/mV)

4: V Unipolar Tip AutoGain (0.9 mm/mV)

Sweep Speed: 25 mm/s

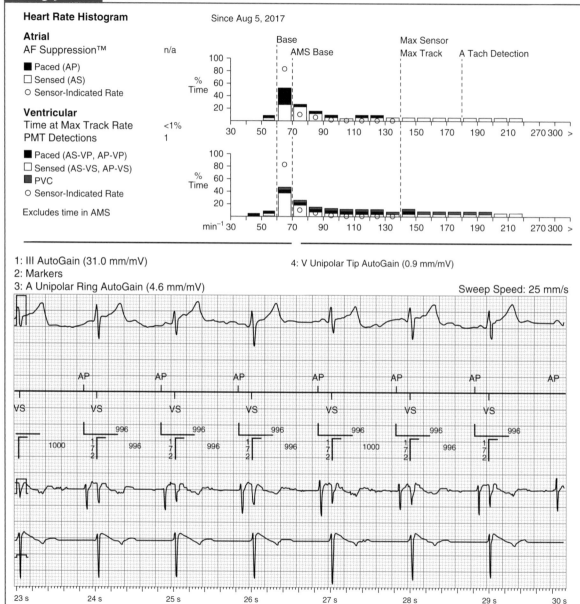

Pacemaker interrogation can also generate a heart rate profile (above) and an ECG using the lead tip and pacemaker generator box as the poles (bottom). This allows both the automated sensing functions of the pacemaker to be checked and some useful diagnostics

The letters of the NBG Code signify the following:

A = right atrium
V = right ventricle
D = dual
0 = none
I = inhibited

In the code:
- the first letter describes the chamber(s) paced (A, V or D)
- the second letter describes the chamber(s) sensed (A, V, D or 0)
- the third letter describes the response to a sensed event (I, D or 0)

- a fourth letter (R) is used when the rate modulation is programmable.

The most commonly used types of pacemaker are listed in Table 5.1.

Right ventricular pacemakers (VVI)

One of the most common types of pacemakers, these have a single lead implanted in the right ventricle, either at the apex (Fig. 5.23) or in a septal position (for example see V-lead position in Fig. 5.35). The septal position has theoretical advantages in enhancing normal synchronized ventricular contraction. The lead senses electrical activity in the right ventricle and, if no spontaneous cardiac activity

TABLE 5.1 Types of Pacemakers

Nomenclature	Chamber(s) with implanted electrode	Device function
Single chamber		
VVI	RV	RV sensed, RV paced Sensed event inhibits pacemaker
AAI	RA	RA sensed, RA paced Sensed event inhibits pacemaker
VVI/ICD	RV	RV sensed, RV paced Sensed event inhibits pacemaker In case of ventricular fibrillation, ICD defibrillates
Dual chamber		
DDD	RA RV	RA and RV sensed, RA and RV paced Sensed event inhibits pacemaker
DDD/ICD	RA – pacing lead RV – pacing and shocking lead	RA and RV sensed, RA and RV paced Sensed event inhibits pacemaker In case of ventricular fibrillation, ICD defibrillates

ICD, implantable cardioverter defibrillator; LA, left atrium; LV, left ventricle; RA, Right atrium; RV, right ventricle.

Fig. 5.23

Right ventricular pacemaker

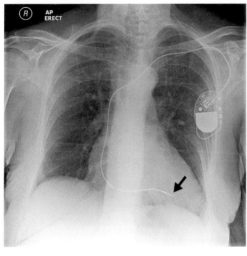

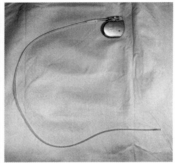

NOTE

- RV pacemaker prior to implantation (right) and chest X-ray showing implantation position (left)
- Pacemaker unit positioned in a subcutaneous pocket beneath the left shoulder
- Pacing lead passing via the subclavian vein, with the lead tip in the conventional right ventricular apical position (arrowed)

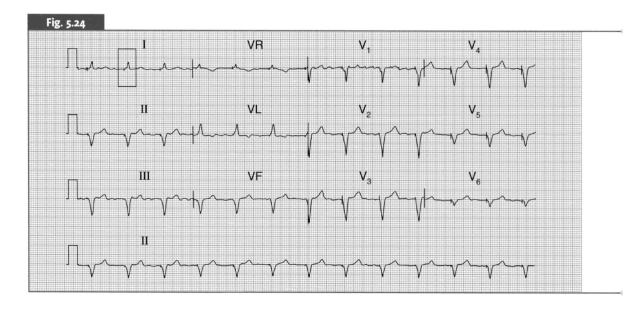

Fig. 5.24

is sensed, paces the ventricle after a predetermined interval. Note that unipolar and bipolar pacing leads cannot be easily differentiated on a routine chest X-ray. The indications for VVI pacing are listed in Box 5.5.

ECG appearance

With bipolar right ventricular pacing, the ECG is characterized by a pacing spike followed by a broad QRS complex of left bundle branch block morphology, because cardiac depolarization originates from the lead tip in the right ventricle (Fig. 5.24). The pacing spikes vary in size and morphology in different ECG leads and in different patients, and may not be visible in all leads.

With unipolar pacing, in which the electrical circuit is between the lead tip and the pacemaker box, the pacing spike is very large compared to that associated with bipolar pacing, in which the poles are close together (Fig. 5.25).

VVI bipolar pacing

NOTE

- Pacing spike followed by a paced ventricular beat with a broad complex. Because the paced complex originates from the right ventricle, its morphology is similar to that seen in left bundle branch block
- The size of the pacing spike varies in different ECG leads, and it may not be visible
- The unchanging morphology of the QRS complex in the rhythm strip confirms continuous right ventricular pacing
- Underlying atrial fibrillation (best seen in lead V_1)

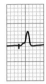

Pacing spike followed by broad QRS complex

BOX 5.5 Indications for VVI Pacing

- Atrial fibrillation with a slow ventricular rate or pauses
- Sinoatrial disease (bradycardia–tachycardia syndrome), in which patients have atrial-driven tachyarrhythmias (such as fast atrial fibrillation) but periods of relative bradycardia that prevent pharmacological rate control
- 'Backup' pacemaker, in patients with occasional pauses due to sinus node disease or atrioventricular block but a predominantly spontaneous cardiac rhythm
- In the very elderly, in whom more sophisticated devices are unlikely to improve function

If the pacemaker senses spontaneous cardiac activity, pacing will be suppressed for a predetermined time interval. The ECG will then show intermittent pacing, with varying amounts of paced ventricular rhythm and underlying ventricular rhythm (Figs 5.26 and 5.27).

The ECGs of patients with pacemakers programmed to provide a backup function for occasional slow rhythms may show no paced beats at all, if the intrinsic cardiac rate exceeds the programmed pacing rate.

The underlying atrial rhythm can be determined from the ECG, and may be important for clinical decisions, such as anticoagulation. There may be sinus rhythm, atrial fibrillation, atrial flutter (Fig. 5.27) or complete block (Fig. 5.28).

Fig. 5.25

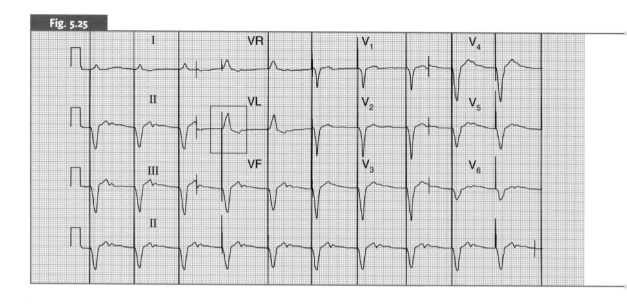

Fig. 5.26

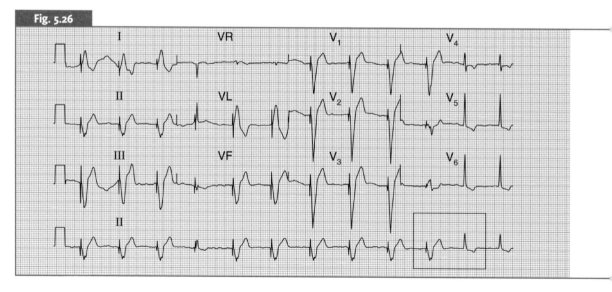

VVI unipolar pacing

NOTE

- Pacing spikes much larger than with bipolar pacing

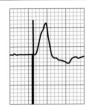

Large ventricular pacing spike

Intermittent VVI pacing

NOTE

- Ventricular pacing
- Underlying rhythm can be seen to be atrial fibrillation
- Final two beats with narrow complexes are not paced – the intrinsic heart rate exceeds that of the pacemaker

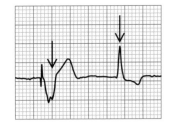

First beat paced, second beat unpaced

Fig. 5.27

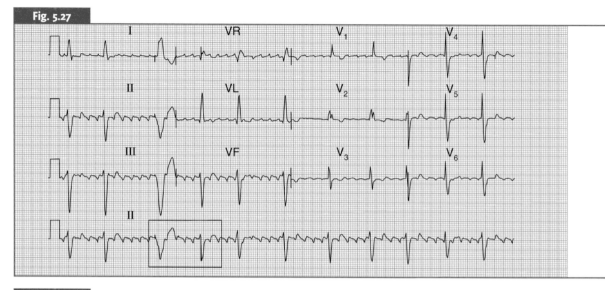

Fig. 5.28

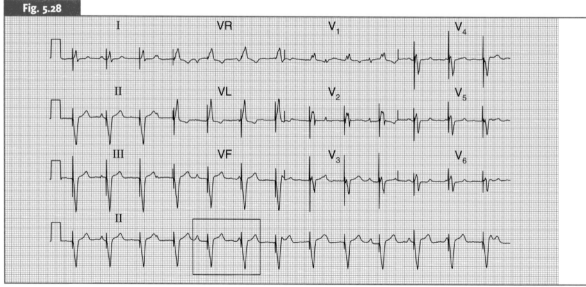

Atrial flutter with intermittent VVI pacing
NOTE
- Underlying atrial flutter with variable block
- After the second beat the subsequent pause exceeds the trigger rate for the pacemaker, and the third beat shows ventricular pacing
- All other QRS complexes are intrinsic (i.e. not paced), indicating normal ventricular sensing
- Vertical lines where the lead changes (e.g. from VL to V_2) must not be confused with pacing spikes

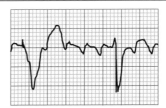

First beat paced, second beat intrinsic

VVI pacing: complete block
NOTE
- Ventricular pacing
- Waves can be seen, unrelated to ventricular beats
- Therefore the underlying rhythm is complete heart block

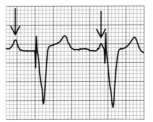

Complete block (P waves arrowed)

Fig. 5.29

Leadless pacemaker

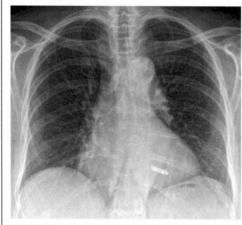

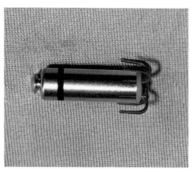

NOTE

- Leadless pacemaker prior to insertion
- Chest X-ray showing post implantation position

Extra functions

Rate response modulation (VVIR) allows an increase in the pacing rate to a preset higher level in the presence of increased activity, as detected from movement. This facilitates some increase in the heart rate with exercise.

Leadless pacemakers

New leadless pacemakers have also been developed (Fig. 5.29). These tether at the right ventricular apex and will generate a similar ECG to a VVI pacemaker.

Fig. 5.30

His pacing system

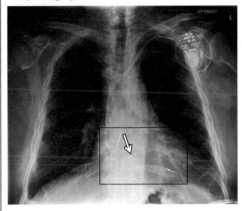

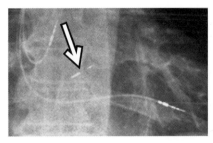

NOTE

- Chest X-ray showing right ventricular pacing lead and right atrial lead (as for a dual chamber pacemaker – see Fig. 5.35) with an additional specialist His pacing lead (white arrow) screwed into the site of the His bundle

His pacemakers

RV apical pacing leads to an inherent reduction in the efficiency of cardiac contraction due to dyssynchronous depolarisation and therefore contraction. A septal lead position can help. New His pacing devices are also being adopted which reduce dyssnchrony by pacing directly into the conducting apparatus of the left ventricle (Figs 5.30, 5.31 and 5.32).

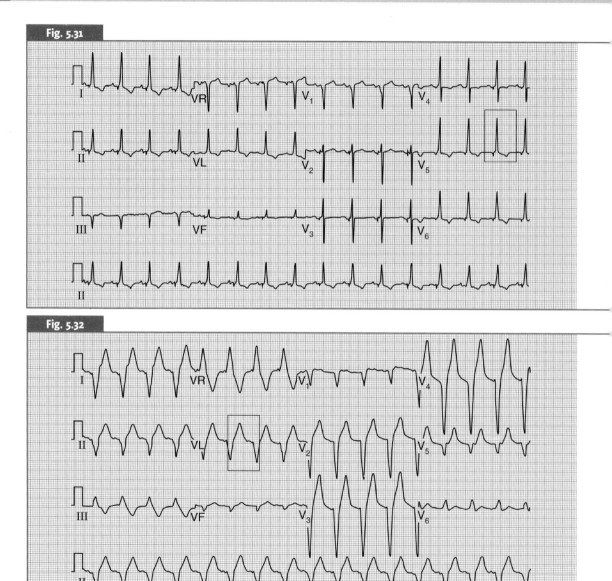

Fig. 5.31

Fig. 5.32

His pacing

NOTE

- Pacing spike following normal P-wave indicating atrial sensing and tracking
- QRS complex following small pacing spike narrow due to pacing directly into the His-purkinje ventricular conducting system

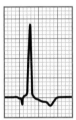

Narrow paced QRS complex

RV apical pacing

NOTE

- Same patient as Fig 5.31 above
- Atrial sensing and tracking
- Very broad QRS complex ventricular depolarisation from RV apical pacing

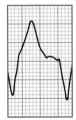

Broad QRS complex with RV apical pacing

Fig. 5.33

Right atrial pacemaker

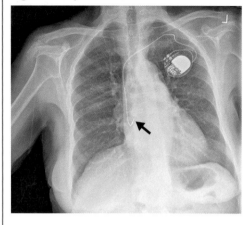

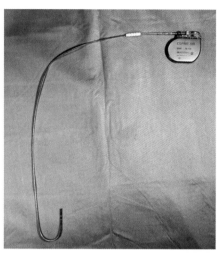

Fig. 5.34

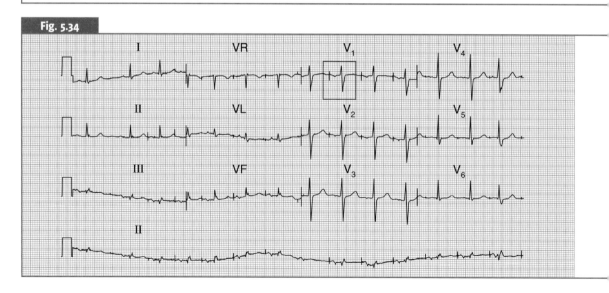

Right atrial pacemakers (AAI)

This is a rarely used mode of pacing, with a single lead implanted in the right atrium, usually in the atrial appendage (Fig. 5.33). This type of pacing senses spontaneous activity in the right atrium, and paces if the sinus node rate falls below a predetermined level.

The indications for AAI pacing are summarized in Box 5.6.

ECG appearance

With atrial pacing the ECG is characterized by a pacing spike followed by a paced P wave. The PR interval and QRS complex are usually normal, indicating no AV node disease (Fig. 5.34).

With intermittent pacing, if the pacemaker senses spontaneous atrial activity, atrial pacing will be suppressed for a predetermined period. Atrial pacemakers are usually implanted to provide backup during fairly rare sinus pauses. Therefore most of the time a normal ECG, with no paced beats, would be expected.

Extra functions

Rate response modulation (AAIR) allows an increase in pacing rate to a preset higher level in the presence of increased activity, as detected from movement. This allows some increase in the heart rate with exercise.

The 'rate drop response' allows the pacemaker to respond to sudden decreases in atrial rate by pacing at a higher rate, and is designed to try to prevent loss of consciousness during episodes of neurocardiogenic syncope.

AAI pacing

NOTE

- Pacing spike precedes each P wave
- The subsequent QRS complex is normal, with no evidence of AV block

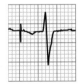

Atrial pacing spike, normal PR interval, normal QRS complex

BOX 5.6 Indications for AAI Pacing

- Sinus node disease with no evidence of atrioventricular node disease
- Young patients with symptomatic sinus pauses

Fig. 5.35

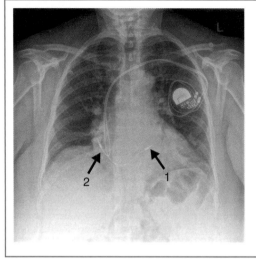
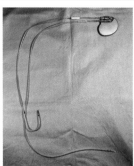

Fig. 5.36

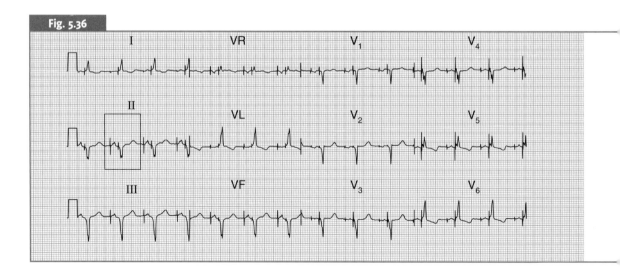

Dual chamber pacemaker

NOTE

- Dual chamber pacemaker prior to implantation (right) and chest X-ray showing implantation position (left)
- Pacemaker unit in the left prepectoral position
- Ventricular lead positioned in right ventricular septal position (arrow 1)
- Atrial lead positioned in this case in the right atrial appendage position arrow 2)

DDD pacing: atrial and ventricular pacing

NOTE

- Continuous atrial and ventricular pacing throughout
- Pacing spikes precede both P waves and QRS complexes

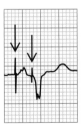

Atrial pacing followed by ventricular pacing in lead II

Dual-chamber pacemakers (DDD)

DDD pacemakers are frequently used devices with two leads, one implanted in the right atrium and one in the right ventricle (Fig. 5.35).

The right atrial and ventricular chambers are both sensed. The atrial pacing lead will pace if no atrial activity is sensed within a predetermined interval. A maximum PR interval is also predetermined. If this is exceeded (following either a spontaneous P wave or a paced P wave) and no ventricular beat is sensed, then the ventricular paced beat is triggered.

Dual-chamber pacing is appropriate with the conditions listed in Box 5.7.

ECG appearance

When both the atrium and the ventricle are being paced, an atrial pacing spike is followed by a paced P wave, then a ventricular pacing spike is followed by a paced ventricular beat (Fig. 5.36).

When the intrinsic atrial rate exceeds the threshold for atrial pacing, 'atrial tracking' occurs. Atrial sensing takes place, but the intrinsic PR interval is longer than the programmed AV delay – leading to ventricular pacing. The ECG shows no atrial pacing spikes, but shows spontaneous P waves followed by ventricular pacing spikes and paced ventricular beats (Fig. 5.37).

BOX 5.7 Indications for Dual-Chamber Pacing

- Mobitz type II second degree heart block
- Third degree heart block
- Bradycardia–tachycardia syndrome

Fig. 5.37

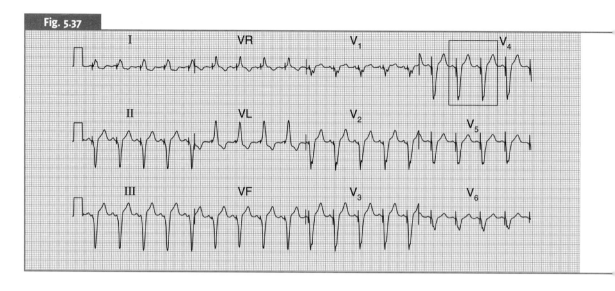

Fig. 5.38

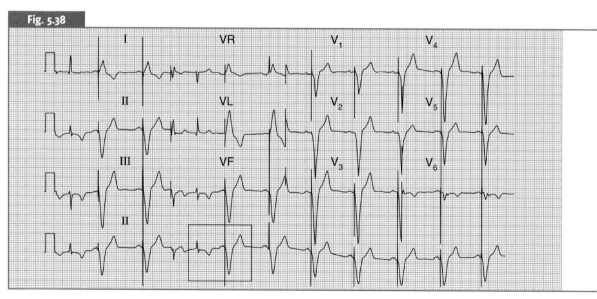

Atrial pacing with ventricular tracking would be an unusual but theoretically possible situation. It would occur if the intrinsic atrial rate was slower than the threshold for atrial pacing, but the PR interval was shorter than the programmed AV delay. Hence there would be atrial pacing and intrinsic QRS complexes. The ECG would show atrial pacing spikes, paced P waves and spontaneous conducted ventricular beats.

In intermittent pacing, spontaneous atrial or ventricular activity will be sensed – leading to the inhibition of pacing in that chamber. If the programmed maximum PR interval is not exceeded, sensed atrial contraction may be followed by an AV conducted beat and a sensed QRS complex. The ECG will then show some intrinsic rhythm and some intermittent pacing (Fig. 5.38).

DDD pacing: atrial tracking
NOTE
- Atrial sensing and ventricular pacing
- Non-paced P waves are followed by ventricular pacing spikes and paced ventricular complexes

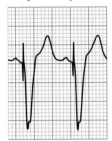

Pacing spike following P wave in lead V₄

DDD pacing: intermittent
NOTE
- Atrial tracking, with atrial sensing and ventricular pacing
- The first, fourth and fifth QRS complexes show the intrinsic underlying rhythm, with appropriate ventricular sensing
- Large pacing spikes are consistent with a unipolar ventricular lead

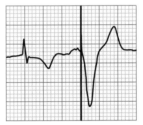

Intrinsic beat followed by a beat showing atrial sensing and ventricular pacing

Specialist functions

Rate response (DDDR) pacing allows an increase in pacing rate to a preset higher level in the presence of increased activity, allowing some increase in the heart rate with exercise.

Anti-atrial-fibrillation algorithms trigger atrial pacing if atrial activity is sensed at a high rate, suggesting the onset of atrial arrhythmia. The aim is to control the atria at a lower rate. In the event of permanent atrial fibrillation, a DDD pacemaker will mode switch to function effectively as a VVI pacemaker.

Abnormal pacemaker function

Pacemaker failure is rare. Most failures are due to problems with the pacing and/or sensing functions of the device. Complete diagnosis will usually require remote interrogation of the pacemaker, by placing over the implanted device a wand or header connected to a specialist programmer. This reveals information about how the device has been performing, as well as assessment of the leads and pacemaker function. There are various potential causes of device failure. Early after implantation, lead displacement may occur (Fig. 5.39). Rarer causes include lead insulation failure or lead fracture (Fig. 5.40). Unexpected battery depletion is rare, because devices are usually monitored regularly.

The investigation of pacemaker malfunction requires specialist techniques and expertise, and the 12-lead ECG can be extremely helpful in showing what has gone wrong.

Failed pacing capture

This occurs when the voltage delivered to the pacemaker lead fails to trigger myocardial depolarization. It is characterized by the presence of pacing spikes

---

Fig. 5.39

Chest X-ray showing right atrial and ventricular lead displacement

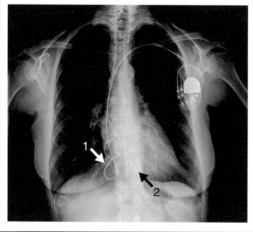

NOTE

- Compare with Fig. 5.35
- The right atrial lead has been displaced from the atrial appendage, to a position much lower in the right atrium (arrow 1)
- The right ventricular lead is looped in the right atrium, with the tip displaced from the apex of the right ventricle (arrow 2)
- Atrial and ventricular pacing and sensing were lost in this patient

but no subsequent atrial or ventricular depolarization (Figs 5.41 and 5.42).

Under-sensing

'Under-sensing' occurs when the device develops an inability to detect intrinsic cardiac activity, and thus fails to suppress pacing in response to an intrinsic beat. The ECG is characterized by the presence of paced and normal beats closer together than would be expected from the programmed interval (Figs 5.43 and 5.44).

Over-sensing or far-field sensing

This arises when sensing occurs in the absence of real intrinsic cardiac activity, triggering the inappropriate suppression of pacing. The ECG is characterized by inappropriately long intervals between beats, when pacing would be expected (Fig. 5.45).

Pacemaker-mediated tachycardia

A rare problem occurs when ventricular pacing triggers retrogradely conducted atrial depolarization, which is then sensed and triggers further ventricular pacing at an inappropriately short interval (Fig. 5.46). Pacemakers have a function for preventing this, called post-ventricular atrial refractory period (PVARP). This is a refractory period after ventricular pacing, in which atrial activity cannot be sensed. Inappropriately rapid pacing will require specialist assessment.

Fig. 5.40

Chest X-ray showing fractured pacing lead

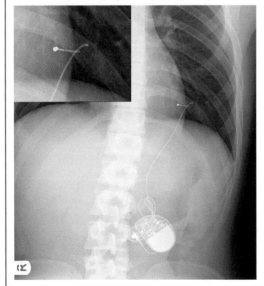

NOTE
- Abdominally placed pacemaker unit (in a child)
- Epicardial lead placed on the epicardial surface of the heart rather than within the right ventricle (endocardial)
- Fracture of the lead just proximal to the lead tip enlarged inset)

Fig. 5.41

Failed pacemaker capture

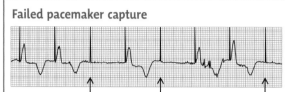

NOTE
- Intermittent failed right ventricular capture – pacing spikes (arrowed) not followed by a QRS complex (VVI pacemaker; no underlying cardiac rhythm)

Fig. 5.42

Failed pacemaker capture

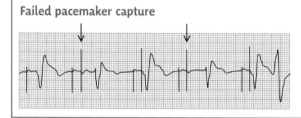

NOTE
- Intermittent failed right ventricular capture (arrowed)
- Ventricular sensing and atrial function appear normal (DDD pacemaker) (Redrawn by permission of Medtronic.)

Fig. 5.43

Pacemaker under-sensing

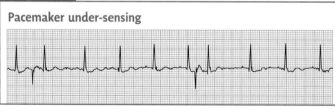

NOTE
- Atrial under-sensing (AAI pacemaker)
- Inappropriate atrial pacing spikes, which capture and conduct from atria to ventricles despite an adequate rate of intrinsic atrial activity – indicating failed atrial sensing

Fig. 5.44

Pacemaker under-sensing

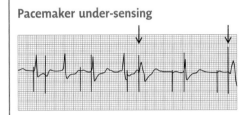

NOTE

- Ventricular under-sensing (DDD pacemaker)
- Atrial and ventricular pacing spikes occur despite an underlying rhythm, indicating failed sensing
- The third and fifth ventricular pacing spikes are normally conducted (arrowed). The remainder form fusion complexes, between the paced and intrinsic QRS complexes (Redrawn by permission of Medtronic.)

Fig. 5.45

Pacemaker over-sensing

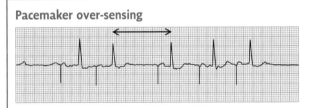

NOTE

- There is an inappropriate gap between the paced atrial and tracked ventricular complexes (arrowed). This could be due to atrial or ventricular over-sensing. In this case, the ventricular lead was at fault. (Redrawn by permission of Medtronic.)

Magnet rate

A simple check of pacemaker function can be made by applying a magnet to the skin over the device. This will trigger obligate pacing at the 'magnet rate' (Fig. 5.47). Pacing spikes will be delivered at this fixed preset rate regardless of the intrinsic rhythm, and should cause depolarization unless delivered at the time of an intrinsic beat, when fusion may occur. The pacemaker will return to normal programmed function when the magnet is removed.

Indications for pacemaker insertion

Table 5.2 summarizes the situations in which permanent pacing is indicated.

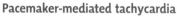

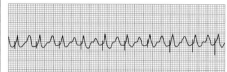

Pacemaker-mediated tachycardia

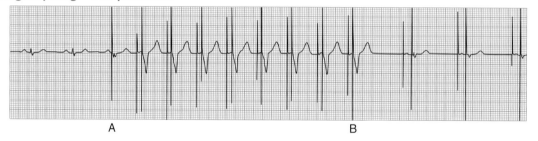

NOTE
- Tachyarrhythmia with pacing spike preceding each QRS complex

Fig. 5.47

Magnet pacing – DDD pacemaker

A   B

NOTE
- Sinus rhythm before magnet application (A)
- Magnet triggers D00 pacing
- Following magnet removal (B), pacing continues until underlying rhythm returns (Redrawn by permission of Medtronic.)

TABLE 5.2 Types of Device and Clinical Indications

Device function	Chamber(s) with implanted electrode	Clinical indications
Single chamber		
VVI	Right ventricle	Slow atrial fibrillation, or atrial fibrillation with pauses 'Backup' with sinus node disease or atrioventricular block Bradycardia–tachycardia syndrome Very elderly patients
AAI	Right atrium	Sinus node disease without atrioventricular block Carotid sinus syncope
VVI/ICD	Right ventricle	**'Primary' prevention** • Heart failure and ejection fraction < 35% and QRS complexes > 120 ms • Heart failure and ejection fraction < 35% and QRS complexes < 120 ms if at high risk of sudden cardiac death • Familial risk of sudden cardiac death including hypertrophic cardiomyopathy, long QT syndrome, Brugada syndrome, or ARVD (arrhythmogenic right ventricular dysplasia) • Surgical repair of congenital heart disease **Secondary prevention** • Survived cardiac arrest due to ventricular fibrillation or VT • Spontaneous sustained VT causing syncope or haemodynamic compromise • Sustained VT and ejection fraction < 35% (but symptoms no worse that NYHA Class III)
Dual chamber		
DDD	Right ventricle Right atrium	Atrioventricular block, usually third degree block or Mobitz type II second degree block Bradycardia–tachycardia syndrome
DDD/ICD	Right ventricle – shocking lead Right atrium – pacing lead	Indications as for VVI/ICD but in patient requiring DDD pacemaker function
Biventricular		
CRT	Right ventricle Left ventricle via coronary sinus ± Right atrium	NYHA Class III* or IV* heart failure and ejection fraction < 35%, plus either left bundle branch block with QRS complexes > 150 ms, or QRS complexes 120 150 ms with echocardiographic dyssynchrony
CRTD	Right ventricle – shocking lead Coronary sinus – left ventricular pacing lead ± Right atrial pacing lead	Indications as for CRT and ICD Patient groups benefiting from combined device not yet clearly defined

*New York Heart Association Functional Classification; Class III/IV indicates moderate/severe heart failure.
Note: CRT with ICD (CRT-D) is indicated for primary prevention in situations where the QRS duration in more prolonged.

The ECG in patients with chest pain

6

History and examination	**195**
Acute chest pain	195
The ECG in the presence of acute chest pain	198
The ECG in patients with myocardial ischaemia	**198**
ECG changes in STEMI	199
ECG changes in NSTEMI	223
The ECG in pulmonary embolism	**231**
The ECG in other causes of chest pain	**235**
Pericarditis	235
ECG pitfalls in the diagnosis of chest pain	**235**
ST elevation	235
R wave changes	237
ST segment and T wave changes	241
Chronic chest pain	244
The investigation of chronic chest pain	245

HISTORY AND EXAMINATION

There are many causes of chest pain. Non-cardiac conditions can mimic a myocardial infarction, and so the ECG can be extremely useful when making a diagnosis. However, as always, the ECG should always be interpreted in its clinical context. The history (including an assessment of coronary risk factors), to a lesser extent the physical examination and other tests including biomarkers of myocardial necrosis, are key to an accurate diagnosis and risk stratification. Some causes of chest pain are listed in Box 6.1.

The ECG in Fig. 6.1 was recorded in an accident and emergency (A&E) department from a 44-year-old man with rather vague chest pain. He was thought to have a viral illness and his ECG was considered to be within normal limits. He was allowed to go home, and died later that day. The post-mortem examination showed a myocardial infarction which was probably a few hours old, and corresponded with his A&E attendance.

Acute chest pain

The features of acute chest pain associated with different causes are summarized in Box 6.2.

The physical examination of a patient with chest pain may reveal nothing other than the signs associated with the pain itself (anxiety, sinus tachycardia, restlessness or a cold and sweaty skin), but some specific signs are worth looking for:
- left ventricular failure suggests myocardial infarction
- a raised jugular venous pressure suggests myocardial infarction or pulmonary embolus

Fig. 6.1

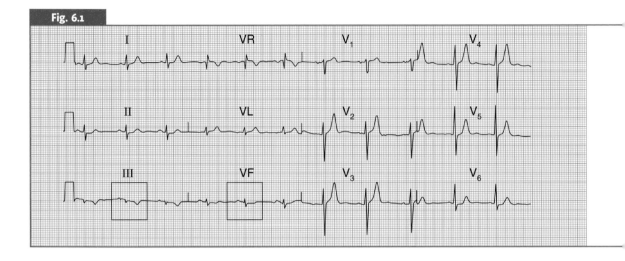

BOX 6.1 Causes of Chest Pain

Acute chest pain
- Myocardial infarction
- Pulmonary embolism
- Pneumothorax
- Other causes of pleuritic pain
- Pericarditis
- Aortic dissection
- Ruptured oesophagus
- Oesophagitis
- Collapsed vertebra
- Herpes zoster

Chronic or recurrent chest pain
- Angina
- Nerve root pain
- Muscular pain
- Oesophageal reflux
- Nonspecific pain

Nonspecific ST segment/T wave changes

NOTE

- Sinus rhythm
- Normal axis
- Normal QRS complexes
- ST segments probably normal, though possibly depressed in leads III and VF
- T wave inverted in lead III (possibly a normal variant) and flattened in VF

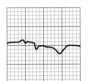

Inverted T wave
in lead III

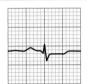

Flattened T wave
in lead VF

BOX 6.2 Features of Acute Chest Pain

Myocardial infarction

- Central
- Radiates to neck, jaw, teeth, arm(s) or back
- Severe
- Associated with nausea, vomiting and sweating
- Not all patients have typical pain, and pain can even be absent

Pulmonary embolism

- Pain similar to myocardial infarction if the embolus is central
- Pleuritic pain if the embolus is peripheral
- Associated with breathlessness or haemoptysis
- Can cause haemodynamic collapse

Other lung disease, e.g. infection or pneumothorax

- Pleuritic
  - worse on breathing
  - often associated with a cough

Pericardial pain

- Can mimic both cardiac ischaemia and pleuritic pain
- Can be recognized because it is relieved by sitting up and leaning forward

Aortic dissection

- Typically causes a 'tearing' pain (as opposed to the 'crushing' sensation of a myocardial infarction)
- Usually radiates to the back

Oesophageal rupture

- Follows vomiting

Spinal pain

- Affected by posture
- Associated root pain follows the nerve root distribution

Shingles (herpes zoster)

- Catches everyone out until the rash appears
- Tenderness of the skin may provide a clue

- a pleural friction rub suggests pulmonary embolism or infection
- a pericardial friction rub suggests pericarditis (viral, secondary to myocardial infarction) or aortic dissection
- aortic regurgitation suggests aortic dissection
- unequal pulses or blood pressure in the arms suggests aortic dissection
- bony tenderness suggests musculoskeletal pain.

The ECG in the presence of acute chest pain

Remember that the ECG can be normal, especially in the early stages of a myocardial infarction. Having said that:

- an abnormal ECG is not necessary to make a diagnosis of myocardial infarction
- an ECG will often (but not always) demonstrate ischaemia in patients with angina *provided that* the patient has pain at the time the ECG is recorded
- with pulmonary embolism there may be classical ECG changes, but these are often not present
- with pericarditis, ECG changes, if present at all, are very nonspecific.

THE ECG IN PATIENTS WITH MYOCARDIAL ISCHAEMIA

Myocardial infarction is, properly, a term describing myocardial cell death due to ischaemia. The histological changes – and ECG changes – can take several hours to appear, and the entire process leading to a healed infarction can take 5 or 6 weeks. Serial ECGs are therefore an important part of the assessment of patients with chest pain. Myocardial injury causes release into the blood of biomarkers including troponin T or I and the MB fraction of creatine kinase (CK-MB). Blood samples should be taken immediately to measure appropriate biomarkers, usually with a high sensitivity troponin assay. However, it is important to remember that plasma biomarker levels take time to rise and the optimal timing of measurements taken to exclude a coronary event depends on the assay used (check with your local laboratory).

Therefore, the release of troponin can reflect the necrosis of myocardial cells; however, it also occurs in situations other than coronary artery occlusion (Box 6.3). Thus, although a rise in the blood levels of troponin supports the diagnosis of myocardial infarction, it is not sufficient, and the most commonly used parts of the 'universal definition' of myocardial infarction require both clinical evidence of myocardial ischaemia and a rise and/or fall of blood troponin levels. Box 6.4 shows the types of infarction listed in the universal definition, drawn up by the ESC/ACCF/AHA/WHF Task Force.*

Acute coronary syndromes are subdivided into those with and without ST segment elevation (ST elevation myocardial infarction [STEMI] and non-ST elevation myocardial infarction [NSTEMI]. These are also referred to sometimes as STE segment elevation ACS (STE-ACS) and non ST segment elevation ACS (NSTE-ACS). The majority of STEMI and some NSTEMI patients develop a rise in troponin, but this may be prevented by very early intervention. Patients with a NSTEMI whose troponin remains normal are classified as having unstable angina. To be as simple as possible, and to avoid confusion, throughout this book we will only describe the relevant ECGs as showing a STEMI or a NSTEMI.

'Stable angina' is an entirely proper diagnostic label for a patient with intermittent chest pain, often on exertion,

---

*Thygesen, K., Alpert, J.S., Jaffe, A.S., et al; ESC Scientific Document Group, Fourth Universal Definition of Myocardial Infarction. *Eur Heart J* (2019), 40, 237–269.

BOX 6.3 Causes of Plasma Troponin Elevation Other Than Myocardial Infarction

- Extreme exertion
- Trauma
- Congestive heart failure (acute or chronic)
- Aortic dissection
- Aortic valve disease
- Hypertrophic cardiomyopathy
- Arrhythmias, including heart block
- Apical ballooning syndrome
- Rhabdomyolysis following cardiac injury
- Pulmonary embolism
- Renal failure
- Stroke; subarachnoid haemorrhage
- Infiltrative diseases (e.g. amyloid, sarcoid)
- Inflammatory diseases – myocarditis and pericarditis
- Drug toxicity
- Critically ill patients with respiratory failure or sepsis
- Burns

BOX 6.4 Criteria for Myocardial Infarction

Acute myocardial infarction

- Detection of rise of cardiac biomarkers (preferably troponin) > 99% of upper reference limit together with evidence of myocardial ischaemia and at least one of the following:
  - symptoms of ischaemia
  - ECG – new changes in ST segments or T waves, or new left bundle branch block
  - development of pathological Q waves
  - imaging evidence of new loss of viable myocardium or new regional wall motion abnormality
- Sudden unexpected cardiac death, often with symptoms and ECG changes of ischaemia; or evidence of fresh coronary thrombus at post mortem, before blood samples are taken or before a rise in cardiac biomarkers could be expected
- Myocardial infarction related to PCI (percutaneous coronary intervention) – a rise of troponin to five times the upper limit of normal, plus new ischaemic symptoms or new ECG changes or imaging evidence of loss of viable myocardium
- Myocardial infarction related to CABG (coronary artery bypass grafting) – elevation of troponin level to 10 times the upper limit of normal, plus either new ECG changes, evidence of loss of viable myocardium, or angiographically demonstrated graft occlusion
- Evidence of imbalance between myocardial oxygen supply and demand unrelated to acute atherothrombosis

Prior myocardial infarction
Any one of the following:
- Pathological Q waves, with or without symptoms
- Imaging evidence of loss of viable myocardium
- Pathological findings of healed or healing infarction

associated with transient 'ischaemic' ECG changes, and 'chest pain of unknown cause' is the best label if no diagnosis has been made.

ECG changes in STEMI

All patients with STEMI should be considered for primary angioplasty or urgent reperfusion therapy where timely percutaneous coronary intervention is not available and should be treated with guideline-recommended medical therapies.

The sequence of features characteristic of STEMI is:
- normal ECG
- ST segment elevation
- development of Q waves
- ST segment returns to the baseline
- T waves become inverted.

The universal definition of STEMI requires new ST segment elevation at the J point (the junction of the S wave and the ST segment) in two contiguous leads, with the cut-off points in leads V_2–V_3 at > 0.2 mV in men or > 0.15 mV in women, and in other leads at > 0.1 mV. The ECG leads that show the changes typical of a myocardial infarction depend on the part of the heart affected.

Inferior infarction

Figs 6.2–6.4 show traces taken from a patient with a typical history of myocardial infarction: on admission to hospital, 3 h later, and 2 days later. The main changes are in the inferior leads: II, III and VF. Here the ST segments are initially raised, but then Q waves appear and the T waves become inverted. Fig. 6.2 includes coronary angiograms

---

Fig. 6.2

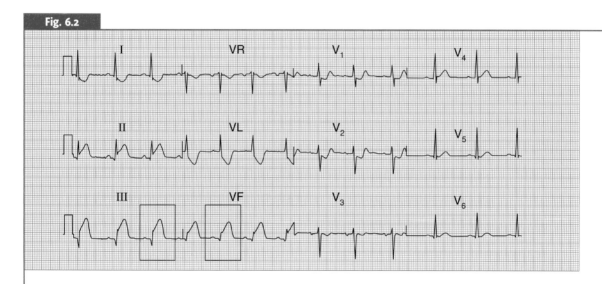

Acute inferior infarction

NOTE
- Sinus rhythm
- Normal axis
- Small Q waves in leads II–III, VF
- Raised ST segments in leads II–III, VF
- Depressed ST segments in leads I, VL, V_2–V_3
- Inverted T waves in leads I, VL, V_3

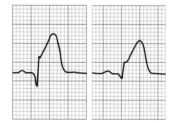

Raised ST segments in leads III and VF

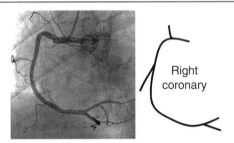

Angiogram showing normal right coronary artery

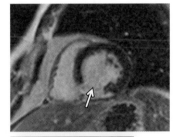

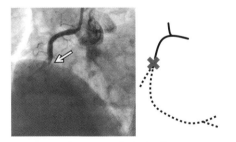

Angiogram showing occluded right coronary artery in inferior STEMI

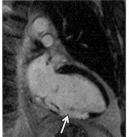

MRI showing established inferior myocardial infarction (white area – arrowed)

Fig. 6.3

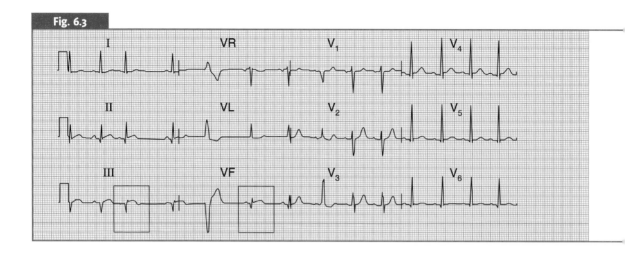

Fig. 6.4

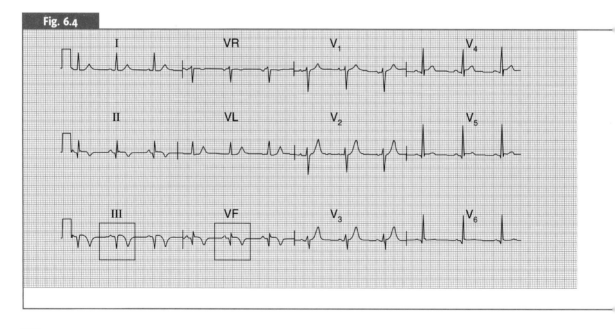

Evolving inferior infarction

NOTE

- Same patient as in Figs 6.2 and 6.4
- Sinus rhythm with ventricular extrasystoles
- Normal axis
- Deeper Q waves in leads II–III, VF
- ST segments returning to normal, but still elevated in inferior leads
- Less ST segment depression in leads I, VL, V₃

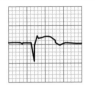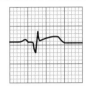

Deeper Q waves in leads III and VF

Evolving inferior infarction

NOTE

- Same patient as in Figs 6.2 and 6.3
- Sinus rhythm
- Normal axis
- Q waves in leads II–III, VF
- ST segments nearly back to normal
- T wave inversion in leads II–III, VF
- Lateral ischaemia has cleared (as shown by ST segments in lateral leads)

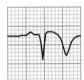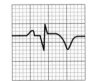

Q waves, normal ST segments, and inverted T waves in leads III and VF

and a cardiac magnetic resonance imaging (MRI) showing the myocardial injury resulting from an occluded right coronary artery in an inferior STEMI.

Anterior and lateral infarction

The changes of anterior infarction are seen in leads V_2–V_5. Lead V_1, which lies over the right ventricle, is seldom affected (see Fig. 6.5, which includes corresponding coronary angiograms and cardiac MRI).

When the lateral wall of the left ventricle is damaged by occlusion of the left circumflex coronary artery, leads I, VL and V_6 will show infarction changes. Fig. 6.6 shows the record of a patient with an acute lateral STEMI, with the corresponding coronary angiograms and cardiac MRI. Fig. 6.7 shows a record taken 3 days after a lateral infarction, with Q waves and inverted T waves in leads I, VL and V_6.

Fig. 6.5

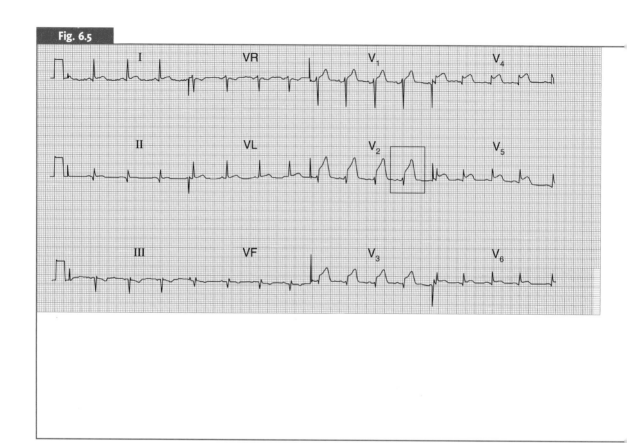

Anterior infarction

NOTE

- Sinus rhythm
- Normal axis
- Raised ST segments in leads V_2–V_5

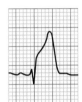

Raised ST segment in lead V_2

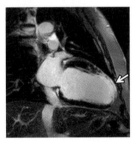

MRI showing established antero-apical myocardial infarction (white area – arrowed)

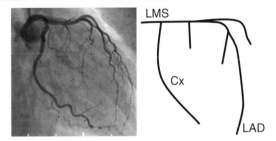

Angiogram showing normal left coronary artery: LMS, left main stem coronary artery; Cx, circumflex branch; LAD, left anterior descending branch

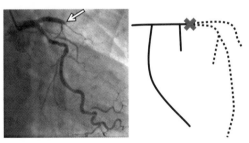

Angiogram showing occluded left anterior descending branch in anterior STEMI

Fig. 6.6

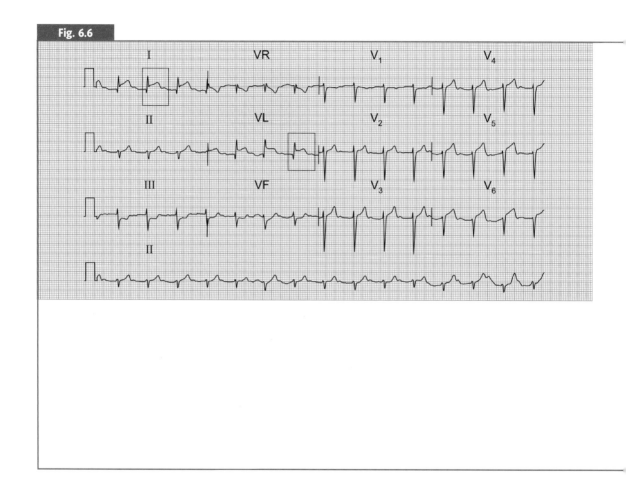

Acute lateral infarction

NOTE

- Sinus rhythm
- First degree block
- Left axis deviation
- Normal axis
- Q waves in leads I, VL
- Raised ST segments in leads I, VL, V_5–V_6

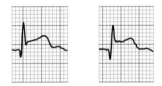

Raised ST segments in leads I and VL STEMI

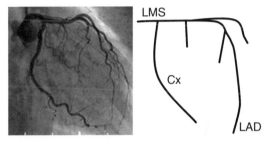

Angiogram showing normal left coronary artery: LMS, left main stem coronary artery; CX, circumflex branch; LAD, left anterior descending branch

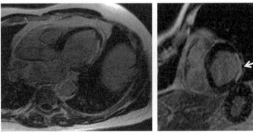

MRI showing established lateral myocardial infarction (white area – arrowed)

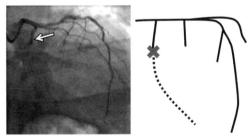

Angiogram showing occluded left circumflex branch in lateral STEMI

Fig. 6.7

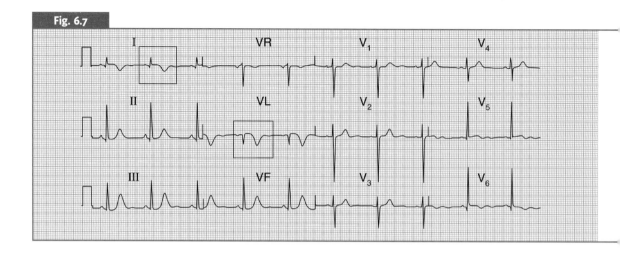

Fig. 6.8

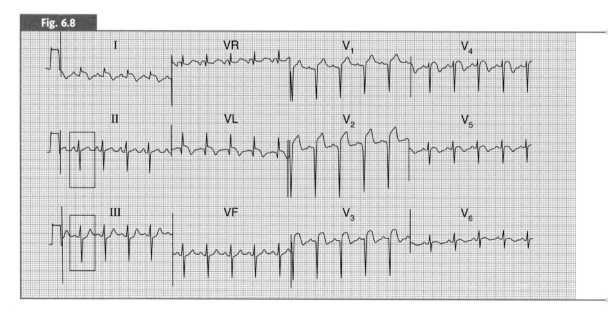

Lateral infarction (after 3 days)

NOTE

- Sinus rhythm
- Normal axis
- Q waves in leads I, VL, V_6 (could be septal)
- ST segments isoelectric
- Inverted T waves in leads I, VL, V_6

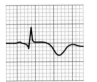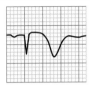

Inverted T waves in leads I and VL

Acute anterolateral infarction with left axis deviation

NOTE

- Sinus rhythm
- Left axis deviation
- ST segments now returning to normal
- T wave inversion in leads I, VL, V_4–V_5

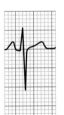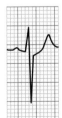

S waves in leads II and III: left axis deviation

The ECG in Fig. 6.8 shows an acute STEMI affecting both the anterior and lateral parts of the left ventricle.

The ECG in Fig. 6.9 was recorded several weeks after an anterolateral myocardial infarction. Although the changes in leads I and VL appear 'old', having an isoelectric ST segment, there is still ST segment elevation in leads V_3–V_5. If the patient had just been admitted to hospital with chest pain these changes would be taken to indicate an acute infarction, but this patient had pain more than a month previously. Persistent ST segment elevation is quite common after an anterior infarction: it sometimes indicates the development of a left ventricular aneurysm, but it is not reliable evidence of this.

An old anterior infarction often causes only what is called 'poor R wave progression'. Fig. 6.10 shows the record from a patient who had had an anterior infarction some years previously. A normal ECG would show a progressive increase in the size of the R wave from lead V_1 to V_5 or V_6 (see p. 19). In this case, the R wave remains

Fig. 6.9

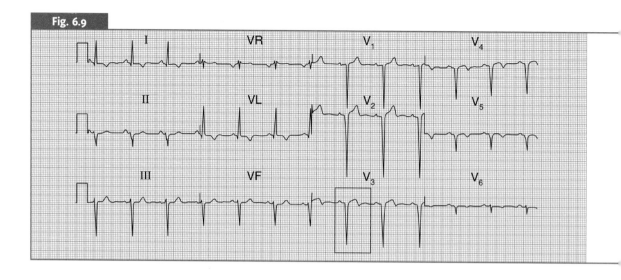

Fig. 6.10

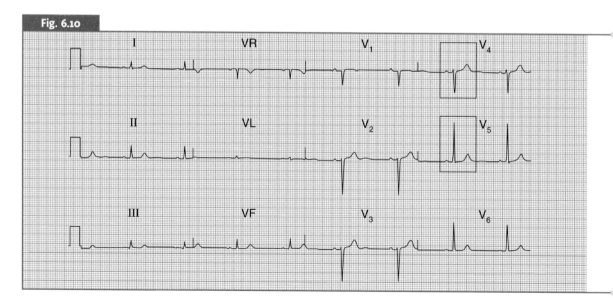

Anterolateral infarction, ?age

NOTE

- Sinus rhythm
- Left axis deviation
- Q waves in leads I–II, V_2–V_5
- Raised ST segments in
- Leads V_3–V_5
- Inverted T waves in leads I, VL, V_4–V_6

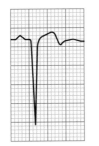

Raised ST segment in lead V_3

Old anterior infarction

NOTE

- Sinus rhythm
- Normal axis
- Small R waves in leads V_3–V_4, large R waves in V_5: this is 'poor R wave progression'

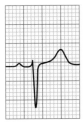

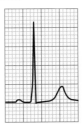

Small R wave in lead V_4

Tall R wave in lead V_5

---

very small in leads V_3 and V_4, but becomes normal-sized in V_5. This loss of R-wave 'progression' indicates the old infarction.

The time taken for the various ECG changes of infarction to occur is extremely variable, and the ECG is an unreliable way of deciding when an infarction occurred. Serial records showing progressive changes are the only way of timing the infarction from the ECG.

Posterior infarction

It is possible to 'look at' the back of the heart by placing the V lead on the back of the left side of the chest, but this is not done routinely because it is inconvenient, and the complexes recorded are often small.

An infarction of the posterior wall of the left ventricle can, however, be detected from the ordinary 12-lead ECG because it causes a dominant R wave in lead V_1. Normally the left ventricle, being more muscular than the right, exerts a greater influence on the ECG, so in lead V_1 the QRS complex is predominantly downward. With a posterior infarction, the rearward-moving electrical forces are lost, so lead V_1 'sees' the unopposed forward-moving depolarization of the right ventricle, and records a predominantly upright QRS complex.

Fig. 6.11 shows the first record from a patient with acute chest pain. There is a dominant R wave in lead V_1 and ischaemic ST segment depression in leads V_2–V_4. The chest electrodes were then moved to the V_7–V_9 positions: all in the same horizontal plane as V_5, with V_7 on the posterior axillary line, V_9 at the edge of the spine, and V_8 halfway between, on the midscapular line. The ECG record then showed raised ST segments, with Q waves typical of an acute infarction.

Fig. 6.11

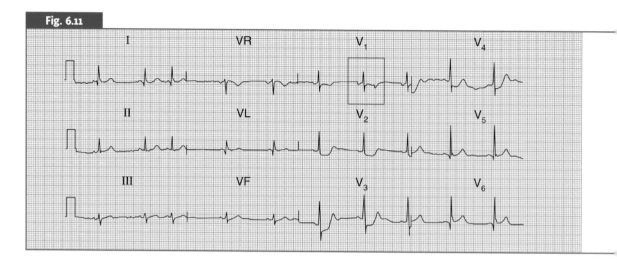

Fig. 6.12

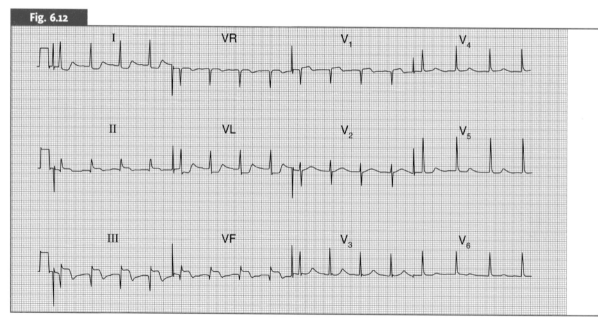

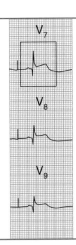

Posterior infarction

NOTE
- Sinus rhythm with atrial extrasystoles
- Normal axis
- Dominant R waves in lead V_1 suggest posterior infarction
- ST segment depression in leads V_2–V_4
- Q waves and ST segment elevation in leads V_7–V_9 (posterior leads)

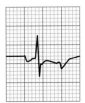

Dominant R wave in lead V_1

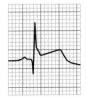

Q wave and raised ST segment in lead V_7

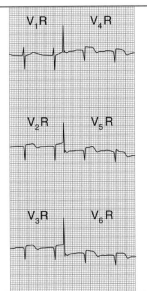

Inferior and right ventricular infarction

NOTE
- Sinus rhythm
- Normal axis
- Raised ST segments in leads II–III, VF
- Raised ST segments in leads V_2R–V_5R
- Q waves in leads III, VF, V_2R–V_6R

Right ventricular infarction

Inferior infarction is sometimes associated with infarction of the right ventricle. Clinically, this is suspected in a patient with an inferior infarction when the lungs are clear but the jugular venous pressure is elevated. The ECG will show raised ST segments in leads recorded from the right side of the heart. The positions of the leads correspond to those on the left side as follows: V_1R is in the normal V_2 position; V_2R is in the normal V_1 position; V_3R, etc. are on the right side, in positions corresponding to V_3, etc. on the left side. Fig. 6.12 is from a patient with an acute right ventricular infarct.

Fig. 6.13

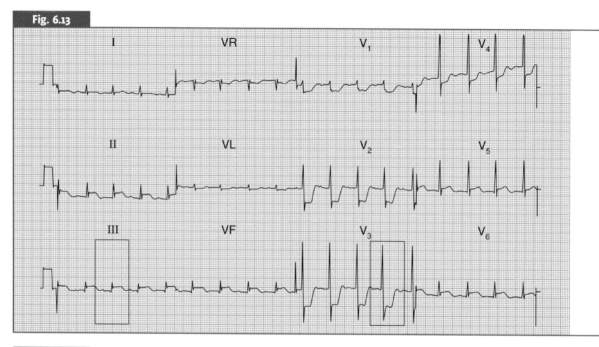

Fig. 6.14

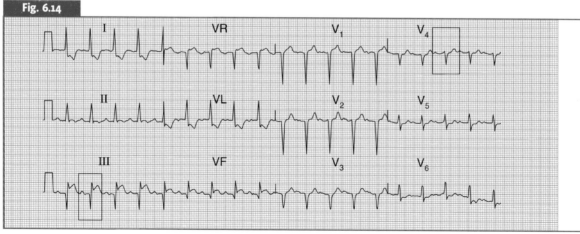

Multiple infarctions

Infarction of more than one part of the left ventricle causes changes in several different ECG territories. This usually implies disease in more than one of the main coronary arteries. The ECG in Fig. 6.13 shows an acute inferior myocardial infarction and marked anterior ST segment depression. Later, coronary angiography showed that this patient had a significant stenosis of the left main coronary artery.

Fig. 6.14 is the record from a patient with an acute inferior myocardial infarction. Poor R wave progression in leads V$_2$–V$_4$ indicates an old anterior infarction as well.

Fig. 6.15 is an ECG showing an acute inferior STEMI and anterior T wave inversion due to an NSTEMI of uncertain age.

Fig. 6.16 is an ECG showing an acute anterior myocardial infarction. Deep Q waves in leads III and VF indicate an old inferior infarction.

Acute inferior infarction and anterior ischaemia
NOTE
- Sinus rhythm
- Normal axis
- Raised ST segments in leads II–III, VF
- ST segment depression in leads V$_1$–V$_4$

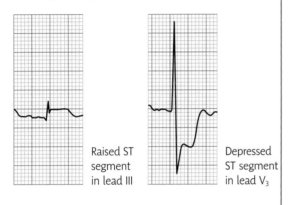

Raised ST segment in lead III

Depressed ST segment in lead V$_3$

Acute inferior and old anterior infarctions
NOTE
- Sinus rhythm
- Normal axis
- Q waves in leads III, VF
- Raised ST segments in leads III, VF
- Poor R wave progression in anterior leads

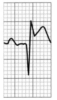 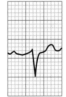

Q wave and raised ST segment in lead III

Loss of R wave in lead V$_4$

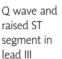

Fig. 6.15

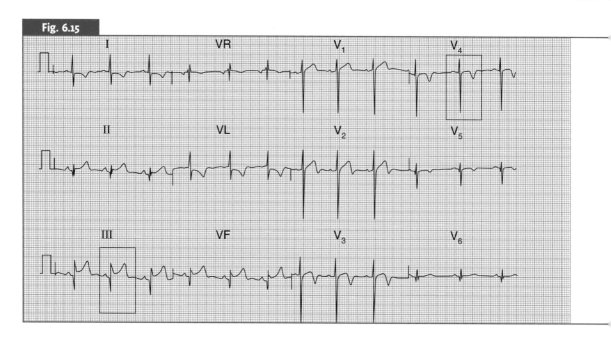

Fig. 6.16

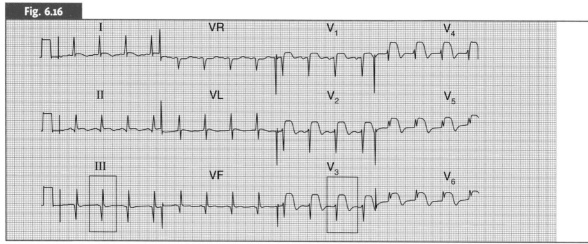

Acute inferior infarction (STEMI) and anterior NSTEMI

NOTE

- Sinus rhythm
- Normal axis
- Q waves in leads II–III, VF
- ST segment elevation in leads II–III, VF
- T wave inversion in leads V_3–V_5

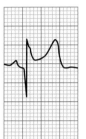 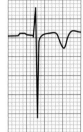

Q wave and ST segment elevation in lead III

Inverted T wave in lead V_6

Acute anterior and old inferior infarctions

NOTE

- Sinus rhythm
- Normal axis
- Q waves in leads II–III, VF
- ST segment elevation in leads V_2–V_6

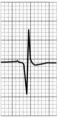 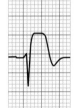

Q wave in lead III

Raised ST segment in lead V_3

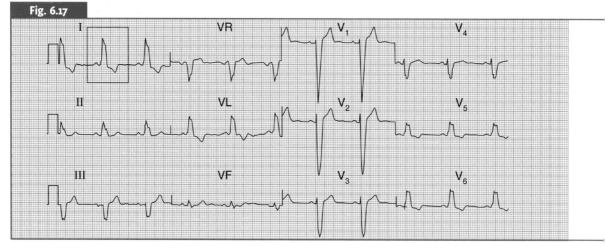

Fig. 6.17

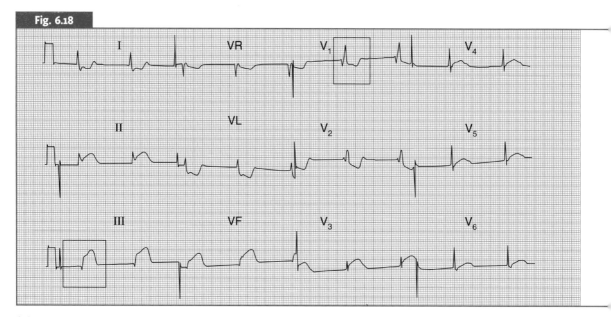

Fig. 6.18

Bundle branch block and myocardial infarction

Left bundle branch block. Left bundle branch block (LBBB) is very rare in patients with totally normal hearts, but it may be associated with many different heart diseases (Box 6.5).

With LBBB, the abnormal and slow conduction into the left ventricle, and the abnormal pattern of repolarization, mean that changes dues to myocardial infarction can be difficult to interpret (Fig. 6.17). However, this does not mean that the ECG can be totally disregarded. If a patient has chest pain that could be ischaemic and the ECG shows LBBB that is known to be new, it can be assumed that an acute infarction has occurred, and appropriate treatment should be given.

Right bundle branch block. Right bundle branch block (RBBB) will not necessarily obscure the pattern of inferior infarction (Fig. 6.18).

Anterior infarction is more difficult to detect, but RBBB does not affect the ST segment and when this is raised in a patient who clinically has had an infarction, the change is probably significant (Fig. 6.19).

ST segment depression associated with RBBB indicates ischaemia (Fig. 6.20). However, T wave inversion in the anterior leads (Fig. 6.21) is more difficult to interpret because it is a common feature of RBBB itself.

Left bundle branch block

NOTE

- Sinus rhythm
- Normal axis
- Wide QRS complexes with LBBB pattern
- Inverted T waves in leads I, VL, V_5–V_6

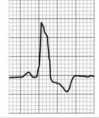

Broad QRS complex and inverted T wave in lead I

Right bundle branch block and acute inferior infarction

NOTE

- Sinus rhythm
- Normal axis
- Wide QRS complex with RSR^1 pattern in lead V_1
- Raised ST segments in leads II–III, VF

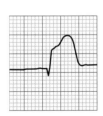

Raised ST segments in lead III

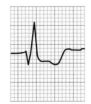

RSR^1 pattern in lead V_1

BOX 6.5 Causes of Left Bundle Branch Block

- Ischaemia
- Hypertension
- Cardiomyopathy
- Myocarditis
- Cardiac channelopathies
- Cardiac tumours
- Sarcoidosis
- Chagas disease
- Operated and unoperated congenital heart disease

Fig. 6.19

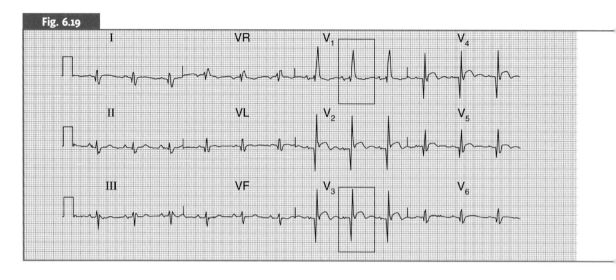

Fig. 6.20

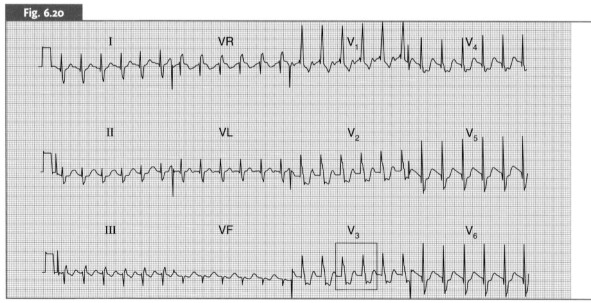

Right bundle branch block and anterior infarction

NOTE

- Sinus rhythm
- Normal axis
- RBBB pattern
- Raised ST segments in leads V_2–V_5

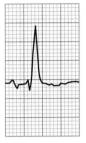

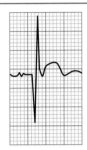

RSR[1] pattern in lead V_1

Raised ST segment in lead V_3

Right bundle branch block and anterior ischaemia

NOTE

- Sinus rhythm
- RBBB pattern
- ST segment depression in leads V_2–V_4

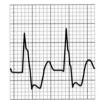

ST segment depression in lead V_3

Fig. 6.21

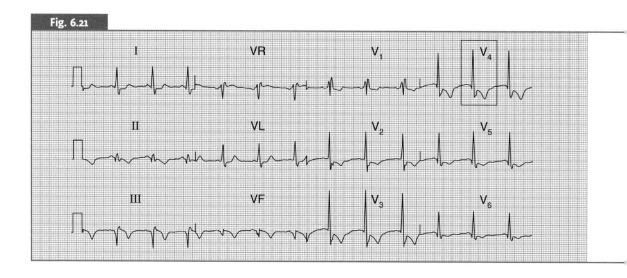

Fig. 6.22

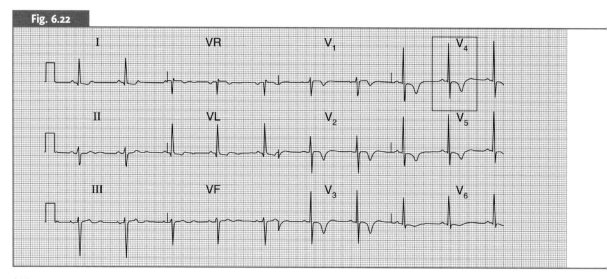

Inferior infarction, right bundle branch block, anterior ischaemia

NOTE
- Sinus rhythm
- Q waves with inverted T waves in leads II–III, VF
- RBBB pattern
- Deep T wave inversion in leads V_3–V_4

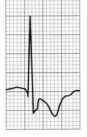

T wave inversion in lead V_4

ECG changes in NSTEMI

All ECG patterns associated with myocardial infarction excluding ST elevation and LBBB are included in this group. This includes infarction causing an abnormality of repolarization that leads to T wave inversion. This pattern is most commonly seen in the anterior and lateral leads (Fig. 6.22).

This ECG pattern used to be called 'subendocardial infarction', but the pathological changes seen in heart muscle after myocardial infarction often do not fit neatly into 'subendocardial' or 'full thickness' patterns. Acute NSTEMI is usually associated with a rise in the blood troponin level. Compared with patients with STEMI, those with NSTEMI have a lower immediate fatality rate but a relatively high risk thereafter, probably reflecting the higher overall burden of vascular disease in this group. All patients with NSTEMI should be considered for inpatient angiography with a view to revascularization as well as optimal medical therapies according to current guidelines.

Anterior non-ST segment elevation acute coronary syndrome (NSTEMI)

NOTE
- Sinus rhythm
- Left axis deviation
- Normal QRS complexes
- Inverted T waves in all chest leads

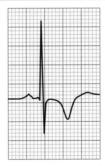

Inverted T wave in lead V_4

Fig. 6.23

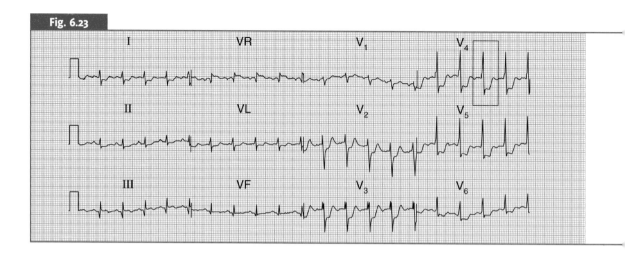

Fig. 6.24

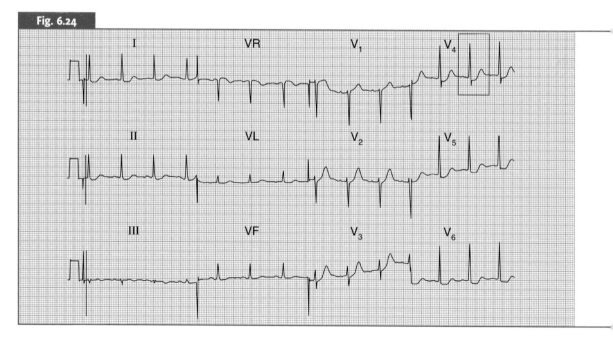

Anterior ischaemia, possible old inferior infarction

NOTE

- Sinus rhythm
- Normal axis
- Small Q waves in leads III, VF
- Inverted T waves in lead III
- Marked ST segment depression in leads V_2–V_6

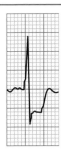

ST segment depression in lead V_4

Anterior ischaemia

NOTE

- Sinus rhythm
- Normal axis
- Normal QRS complexes
- ST segment depression in leads V_4–V_6

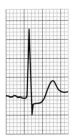

ST segment depression in lead V_4

Ischaemia without myocardial infarction

ECG changes with myocardial ischaemia are variable. Classically cardiac ischaemia causes horizontal ST segment depression; to be diagnostic of ischaemia, there must be horizontal or downward-sloping depression of > 0.05 mV in two contiguous leads, and/or T wave inversion of > 0.1 mV in two contiguous leads. Such changes appear and disappear with the pain of stable angina. Persistent pain and ST segment depression (Fig. 6.23) may not always be associated with a rise in troponin level, although this is uncommon with modern high sensitivity troponin assays.

If a patient has chest pain that persists long enough to seek hospital admission, and the ECG shows ST segment depression, this is a high-risk scenario. (Figs 6.24 and 6.25). These patients usually need urgent investigation with a view to coronary revascularization.

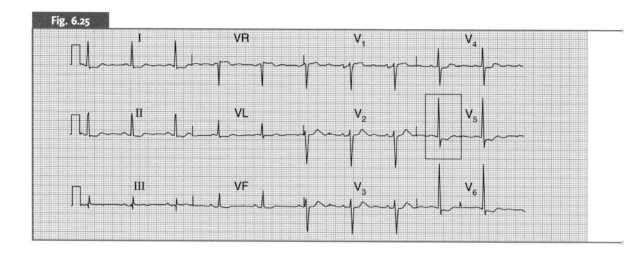

Fig. 6.25

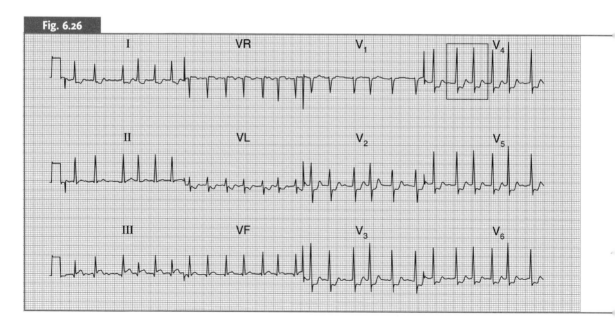

Fig. 6.26

Anterolateral ischaemia

NOTE

- Sinus rhythm
- Possible left atrial hypertrophy (bifid P wave in lead I)
- Normal axis
- Normal QRS complexes
- ST segment depression in leads I, II, V_4–V_6

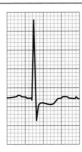

ST segment depression in lead V_5

Atrial fibrillation and anterior ischaemia

NOTE

- Atrial fibrillation, ventricular rate about 130 bpm
- Normal axis
- Normal QRS complexes
- ST segment depression in leads V_2–V_6

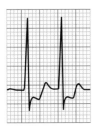

ST segment depression in lead V_4

Ischaemia may be precipitated by an arrhythmia, and will be resolved when either the heart rate is controlled or the arrhythmia is corrected. The ECG in Fig. 6.26 shows ischaemia during atrial fibrillation with a rapid ventricular rate (this patient had not been treated with digoxin). The ECG in Fig. 6.27 shows ischaemic ST segment depression in a patient with an AV nodal re-entry tachycardia and a ventricular rate of > 200 bpm.

Fig. 6.27

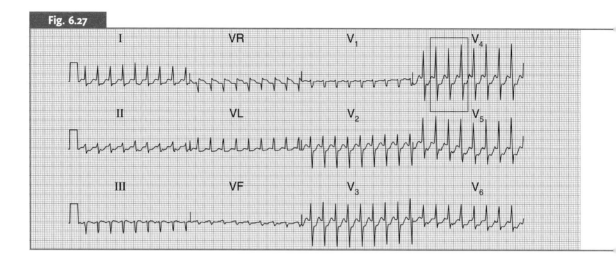

Fig. 6.27

Prinzmetal's variant angina

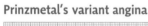

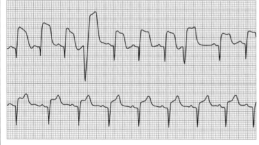

NOTE

- Continuous record
- Initially, the patient had pain, and the ST segment was raised
- The fourth beat is probably a ventricular extrasystole
- As the patient's pain settled, the ST segment returned to normal

AV nodal re-entry tachycardia with anterior ischaemia

NOTE

- Regular narrow complex tachycardia, rate 215 bpm
- No P waves
- ST segment depression in leads V_2–V_6

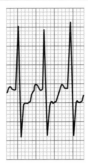

Narrow complexes and ST segment depression in lead V_4

Prinzmetal's 'variant' angina

Angina can occur at rest due to spasm of the coronary arteries. This is accompanied by elevation rather than depression of the ST segments. The ECG appearance is similar to that of an acute ischaemia or myocardial infarction, but the ST segment returns to normal as the pain settles (Fig. 6.28) and coronary angiography is normal. This ECG appearance was first described by Prinzmetal, and it is sometimes called 'variant' angina. Coronary spasm can also rarely be provoked by drugs including recreational cocaine use.

Fig. 6.29

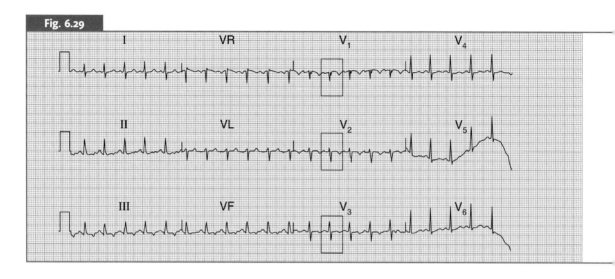

Fig. 6.30

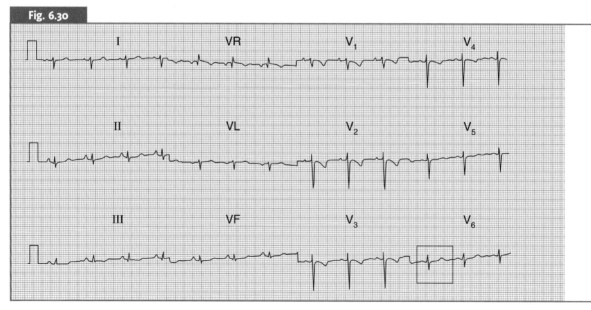

Pulmonary embolus

NOTE

- Sinus rhythm, 130 bpm
- Normal axis
- Normal QRS complexes
- Inverted T wave in leads V_1–V_3, VF

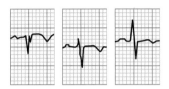

Inverted T wave in leads V_1–V_3

Pulmonary embolus

NOTE

- Sinus rhythm
- Right axis deviation
- Persistent S wave in lead V_6
- T wave inversion in leads V_1–V_4

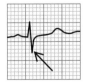

Persistent S wave in lead V_6

THE ECG IN PULMONARY EMBOLISM

Most patients with a pulmonary embolus will have sinus tachycardia, but an otherwise normal ECG.

The ECG abnormalities that may occur in pulmonary embolism are those associated with right ventricular problems:

- peaked P waves
- right axis deviation
- dominant R wave in lead V_1
- inverted T waves in leads V_1–V_3, and sometimes V_4
- RBBB pattern
- shift in the transition point from leads V_3–V_4 to V_5–V_6, leading to a persistent deep S wave in lead V_6
- Q wave and inverted T wave in lead III.

Supraventricular arrhythmias, especially atrial fibrillation, may also occur. There is no particular sequence in which these changes develop, and they can be seen in any combination. The full ECG pattern of right ventricular hypertrophy (right axis deviation, dominant R waves in lead V_1; inverted T waves in leads V_1–V_4, and persistent S waves in lead V_6) is usually only seen in patients with long-standing thromboembolic pulmonary hypertension.

Figs 6.29–6.32 show the records from four patients with a pulmonary embolus – but remember, in most patients the ECG is normal or just shows a sinus tachycardia.

Fig. 6.31

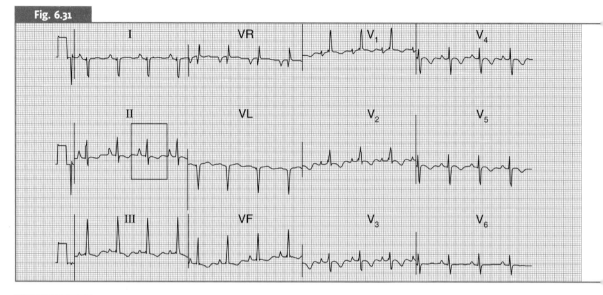

Fig. 6.32

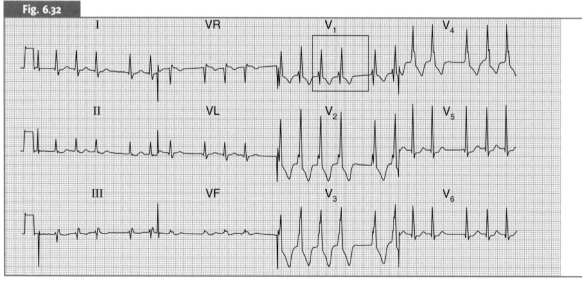

Pulmonary embolus

NOTE

- Sinus rhythm
- Peaked P wave suggests right atrial hypertrophy
- Right axis deviation
- Right bundle branch block pattern
- Persistent S wave in lead V_6
- T wave inversion in leads V_1–V_4

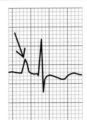

Peaked P wave in lead II

Pulmonary embolus

NOTE

- Atrial fibrillation
- Right bundle branch block pattern

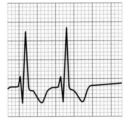

RSR[1] pattern in lead V_1

Fig. 6.33

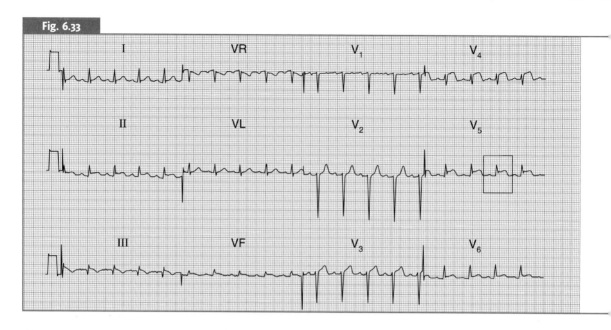

Fig. 6.34

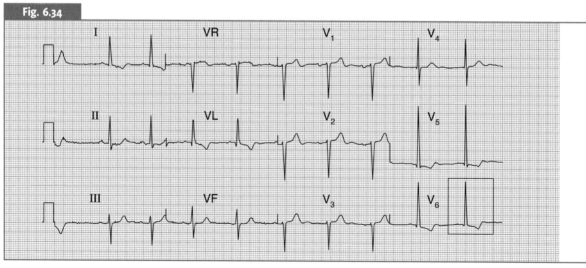

THE ECG IN OTHER CAUSES OF CHEST PAIN

Pericarditis

Pericarditis classically causes 'scalloped' raised ST segments in most leads, sometimes with PR interval depression (Fig. 6.33). This may suggest a widespread acute infarction, but in pericarditis the ST segment remains elevated and Q waves do not develop. This pattern is actually very rare: most patients with pericarditis have either a normal ECG, or a variety of nonspecific ST segment/T wave changes.

Aortic stenosis

Aortic stenosis is an important cause of angina. The ECG should show left ventricular hypertrophy (Fig. 6.34). However, the ECG is an unreliable guide to left ventricular hypertrophy, and the difficulty of distinguishing it from ischaemia is discussed in Ch. 7, p. 265.

ECG PITFALLS IN THE DIAGNOSIS OF CHEST PAIN

The normal variants of the ECG have been described in Chapter 1. The important features that may cause confusion with ischaemia are:

- septal Q waves (mainly in leads II, VL, V_6)
- Q waves in lead III but not VF
- anterior T wave inversion (not uncommon in lead V_2, common in black people in leads V_2, V_3 and sometimes V_4)
- high take-off ST segments.

ST elevation

Several abnormal ECG patterns may cause difficulty in making a diagnosis in patients with chest pain, and some of these are summarized in Table 6.1. Causes of a 'false positive' diagnosis of STEMI include benign early repolarization, LBBB, the Brugada syndrome, myocarditis and

Pericarditis
NOTE
- Sinus rhythm
- Normal axis
- Normal QRS complexes
- ST segment elevation in leads I–III, VF, V_3–V_6

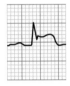

ST segment elevation in lead V_5

Left ventricular hypertrophy
NOTE
- Sinus rhythm
- Tall R waves in leads V_5–V_6
- Inverted T waves in lateral leads

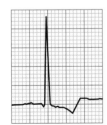

Tall R wave and inverted T wave in lead V_6

235

TABLE 6.1 ECG Pitfalls in the Diagnosis of Chest Pain

Condition	ECG pattern	May be confused with
Normal record	Q waves in lead III but not VF	Inferior infarction
	T wave inversion in leads V_1–V_3 (especially in black people)	Anterior infarction
Left ventricular hypertrophy	T wave inversion in lateral leads	Ischaemia
Right ventricular hypertrophy	Dominant R waves in lead V_1	Posterior infarction
	Inverted T waves in leads V_1–V_3	Anterior infarction
Wolff–Parkinson–White syndrome	Inverted T waves in leads V_2–V_5	Anterior infarction
Hypertrophic cardiomyopathy	T wave inversion in leads V_2–V_5	Anterior infarction
Subarachnoid haemorrhage	T wave inversion in any leads	Ischaemia
Digoxin effect	Downward-sloping ST segment depression or T wave inversion, especially in leads V_5–V_6	Ischaemia

Fig. 6.35

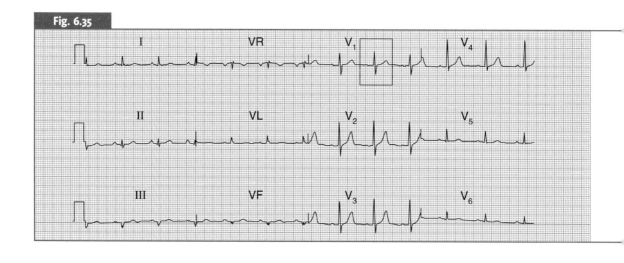

BOX 6.6 ECG Pitfalls in Diagnosing Myocardial Infarction

False positives
- Early repolarization
- Left bundle branch block
- Pre-excitation
- J point elevation syndromes, e.g. Brugada syndrome
- Pericarditis, myocarditis
- Pulmonary embolism
- Subarachnoid haemorrhage
- Metabolic disturbances, e.g. hyperkalaemia
- Cardiomyopathy

- Lead transposition
- Cholecystitis
- Malposition of precordial ECG electrodes
- Tricyclic antidepressants or phenothiazines

False negatives
- Prior myocardial infarction with Q waves and/or persistent ST segment elevation
- Right ventricular pacing
- Left bundle branch block

Old posterior infarction

NOTE
- Sinus rhythm
- Normal axis
- Dominant R waves in leads V_1–V_2
- No other abnormalities

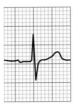

Dominant R wave in lead V_1

pericarditis, and pulmonary embolism. 'False negatives' may be the result of prior myocardial infarction with persistent ST segment elevation, a permanent pacemaker, or LBBB. The conditions in which the ECG can give false positive or false negative results in the diagnosis of myocardial infarction are listed in Box 6.6.

R wave changes

The ECG in Fig. 6.35 shows a dominant R wave in lead V_1. This might be due to right ventricular hypertrophy or to a posterior infarction. Occasionally, it could be a normal variant. Here, the normal axis goes against a diagnosis of right ventricular hypertrophy, and a review of previous ECGs from the patient showed that the dominant R wave was due to a posterior infarction.

The ECG in Fig. 6.36 also shows a dominant R wave in lead V_1. In a patient with chest pain, a posterior infarction

Fig. 6.36

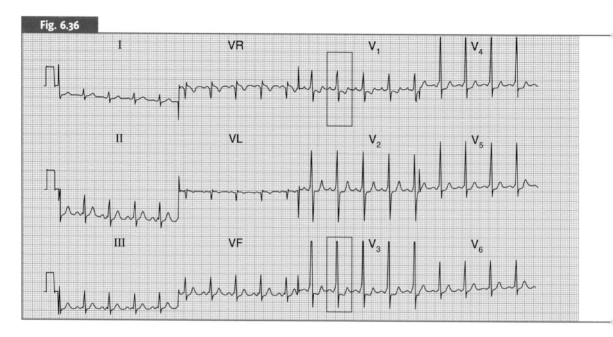

Fig. 6.37

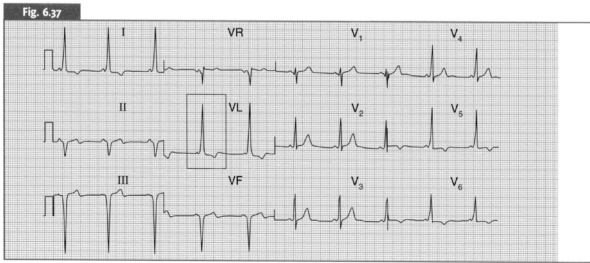

The Wolff–Parkinson–White syndrome type A

NOTE

- Sinus rhythm
- Short PR interval
- Slurred upstroke to QRS complexes
- Dominant R wave in lead V_1: the WPW syndrome type A

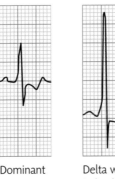

Dominant
R wave in
lead V_1

Delta wave
in lead V_3

The Wolff–Parkinson–White syndrome type B

NOTE

- Sinus rhythm
- Short PR interval
- Left axis deviation
- Delta wave
- Inverted T waves in leads I, VL, V_5–V_6
- No dominant R wave in lead V_1 (the WPW syndrome type B)

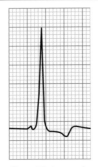

Short PR interval and delta wave in lead VL

Fig. 6.38

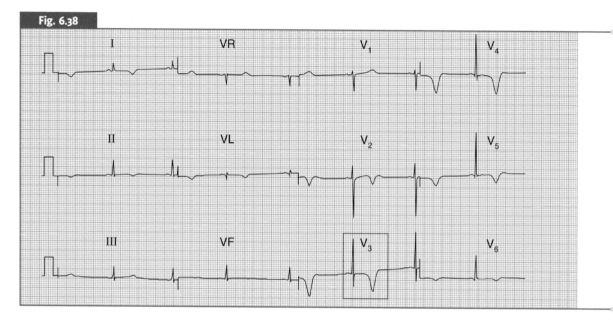

Fig. 6.39

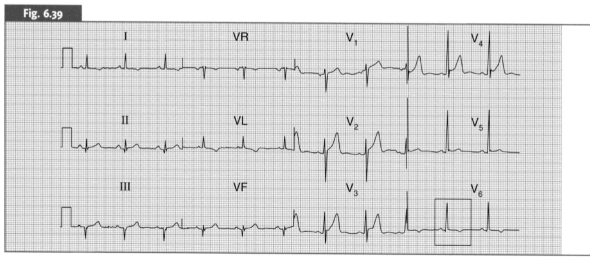

Unexplained T wave abnormality

NOTE

- Sinus rhythm
- Normal axis
- Normal QRS complexes
- QT interval 600 ms
- T wave inversion in leads I–II, VL, V_2–V_6

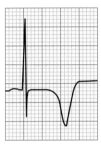

Long QT interval and inverted T wave in lead V_3

Left ventricular hypertrophy

NOTE

- Sinus rhythm
- Normal axis
- Height of R wave in lead V_5 + depth of S wave in lead V_2 = 37 mm
- High take-off ST segment in lead V_4
- T wave inversion in leads I, VL, V_6

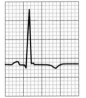

Inverted T wave in lead V_6

might again be considered. However, the PR interval is short and there is a delta wave, so this shows the Wolff–Parkinson–White (WPW) syndrome.

ST segment and T wave changes

It is, however, repolarization (T wave) changes that cause most problems. The lateral T wave inversion in the ECG in Fig. 6.37 might suggest ischaemia, but again this is the WPW syndrome, in which repolarization abnormalities are common.

The anterior and lateral T wave inversion in the ECG in Fig. 6.38 suggests either an NSTEMI or hypertrophic cardiomyopathy. This particular patient was white and asymptomatic, and had no family history of arrhythmias or any cardiac disease. There was no echocardiographic evidence of cardiomyopathy, and coronary angiography was normal. The ECG reverted to normal on exercise, and the T wave inversion and the long QT interval remained unexplained.

Differentiation between lateral ischaemia and left ventricular hypertrophy on the ECG is extremely difficult. The ECG in Fig. 6.39 shows lateral T wave inversion. There are small Q waves in leads III and VF, suggesting a possible old inferior infarction, and the QRS complexes in the chest leads are not particularly tall. Nevertheless, in this patient the lateral T wave inversion was due to left ventricular hypertrophy.

The patient whose ECG is shown in Fig. 6.40 had mild hypertension. The QRS complexes are tall (see Ch. 7, p. 259) and there is lateral T wave inversion, suggesting left ventricular hypertrophy. However, there is also T wave inversion in leads V_3 and V_4, which is unusual in left ventricular hypertrophy. This patient had severe narrowing of the left main coronary artery.

Digoxin therapy causes downward-sloping ST segment depression and T wave inversion (see Ch. 8, p. 303), particularly in the lateral leads, as is seen in Fig. 6.41. The fact that the rhythm is atrial fibrillation with a controlled ventricular rate suggests that the patient is being treated with digoxin.

Fig. 6.40

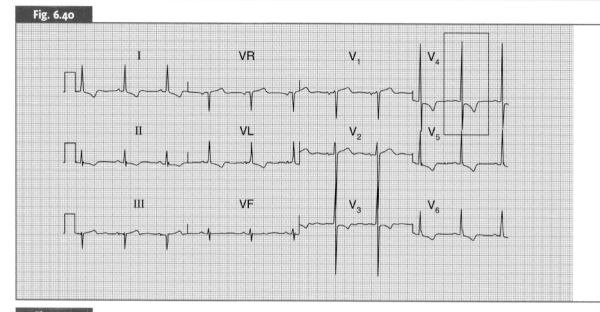

Fig. 6.41

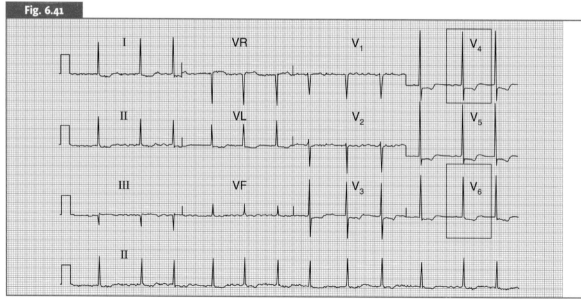

Old anterolateral NSTEMI

NOTE

- Sinus rhythm
- Normal axis
- Tall QRS complexes
- T wave inversion in leads I, VL, V_3–V_6, but this is more marked in lead V_4 than in V_6

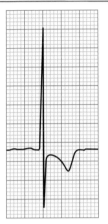

Inverted T wave in lead V_4

Digoxin effect and ischaemia

NOTE

- Atrial fibrillation
- Normal axis
- Normal QRS complexes
- Horizontal ST segment depression in lead V_4
- Downward-sloping ST segment in lead V_6
- Inverted T waves in leads V_3–V_4

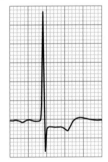

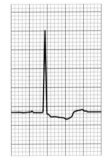

Horizontal ST segment in lead V_4

Downward-sloping ST segment in lead V_6

Fig. 6.42

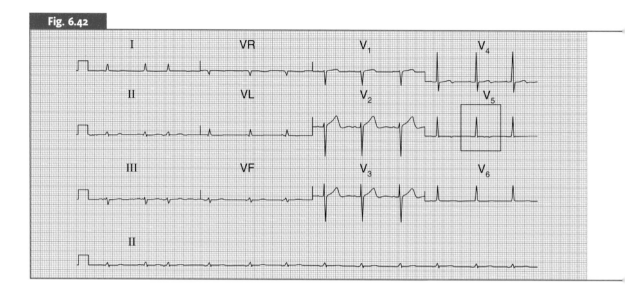

However, T wave inversion in leads V_3 and V_4 is much more likely to be due to ischaemia, as was the case here.

An extremely common finding on the ECG is 'nonspecific T wave flattening' (Fig. 6.42). When a patient is completely well and the heart is clinically normal, this is of no importance. However, in a patient with chest pain that appears to be cardiac, 'nonspecific' ST segment/T wave changes may indicate ischaemia.

Chronic chest pain

The main differential diagnosis of chronic chest pain is between angina and non-cardiac chest pain. Some of these pains are musculoskeletal but in most cases the best diagnostic label is 'chest pain of unknown cause'. This indicates a possible need for later re-evaluation.

The important features in the history that point to a diagnosis of angina are that the pain:

- is predictable
- usually occurs after a constant amount of exercise
- is worse in cold or windy weather
- is induced by emotional stress
- is induced by sexual intercourse
- is relieved by rest, and rapidly relieved by a short-acting nitrate.

The physical signs to look for are:
- evidence of risk factors (high blood pressure, cholesterol deposits, signs of smoking)
- any signs of cardiac disease (aortic stenosis, an enlarged heart, signs of heart failure)
- anaemia (which will exacerbate myocardial ischaemia)
- signs of peripheral vascular disease (which would suggest that coronary disease is also present).

Nonspecific T wave flattening

NOTE

- Recorded at half sensitivity
- Sinus rhythm with supraventricular extrasystoles
- Normal QRS complexes
- Flat T waves in leads I, VL, V_5–V_6

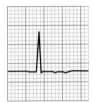

Flat T wave in lead V_5

The investigation of chronic chest pain

The low sensitivity and specificity of exercise testing has greatly reduced its use as a primary diagnostic test for the investigation of chronic chest pain. Imaging investigations such as computed tomography (CT) coronary angiography (including CT-FFR [coronary CT with computational modeling of fractional flow reserve], a technique to derive measures of the functional significance of coronary stenotic disease defined by CT), cardiac stress MRI and myocardial perfusion scintigraphy are increasingly used in accordance with current guidelines. However, exercise testing is still used in centres where these imaging tests are not readily available.

Practical aspects of exercise testing

Reproducible exercise testing needs either a bicycle ergometer or a treadmill. In either case, the exercise should begin at a low level that the patient finds easy, and should be made progressively more difficult. On a bicycle, the pedal speed should be kept constant and the workload increased in steps of 25 W. On a treadmill, both the slope and the speed can be changed and the protocol evolved by Bruce (Table 6.2) is the one most commonly used.

TABLE 6.2 Bruce Protocol for Exercise Testing Using a Treadmill, 3 min at Each Stage

Stage	Speed		Slope		METS (metabolic equivalents)
	Miles per hour	Kilometres per hour	Grade (%)	Degrees to horizontal	
Low level					
01	1.7	2.7	0	0	2.9
02	1.7	2.7	5	2.9	3.7
Standard Bruce protocol					
1	1.7	2.7	10	5.7	5.0
2	2.5	4.0	12	6.8	5.0
3	3.4	5.5	14	8.0	9.5
4	4.2	6.8	16	9.1	13.5
5	5.0	8.0	18	10.2	17.0

Activity	METS
Cleaning floors	4.0
Gardening	4.0
Sexual intercourse	5.0
Bed making	5.0–6.0
Carrying a medium suitcase	7.0

The workload achieved by a patient on a treadmill is sometimes expressed as metabolic equivalents (METS). The rate at which oxygen is used by an average person at rest is 1 MET, and it is equal to 3.5 ml/kg/min. However, few people are average, and oxygen consumption is dependent on weight, age and gender, so METS are not particularly useful. Box 6.7 shows the estimated work-loads imposed by various activities, and hence how exer-cise tolerance (as measured on the treadmill) indicates what a patient might be expected to achieve.

A 12-lead ECG, the heart rate and the blood pressure should be recorded at the end of each exercise period. The maximum heart rate and blood pressure are in some ways more important than the maximum workload achieved, because the latter is markedly influenced by physical fitness. However, interpreting the ECG recorded during exercise testing is difficult when the baseline ECG is abnormal or the patient is taking drugs which reduce heart rate and alternative investigations should be consid-ered. This includes in cases of:
- bundle branch block
- ventricular hypertrophy
- WPW syndrome
- digoxin therapy
- beta-blocker therapy.

Reasons for discontinuing an exercise test

1. At the request of the patient – because of pain, breathlessness, fatigue or dizziness.

2. If the systolic blood pressure begins to fall. Normally, systolic pressure will rise progressively with increasing exercise level, but in any subject a point will be reached at which systolic pressure reaches a plateau and then starts to fall. A fall of 10 mmHg is an indication that the heart is not pumping effectively and the test should be stopped – if it is continued, the patient will become dizzy and may fall. In healthy subjects, a fall in systolic pressure is seen only at high workloads, but in patients with severe heart disease the systolic pressure may fail to rise on exercise. The amount of exercise the patient can carry out before the systolic pressure falls is thus a useful indicator of the severity of any heart disease.

3. It is conventional to discontinue the test if the heart rate increases to 80% of the predicted maximum for the patient's age. This maximum can be calculated in beats/min by subtracting the patient's age in years from 220. Patients with severe heart disease will usually fail to attain 80% of their predicted maximum heart rate, and the peak rate is another useful indicator of the state of the patient's heart. It is, of course, important to take note of any treatment the patient may be receiving, because a beta-blocker will prevent the normal increase in heart rate.

4. Exercise should be discontinued immediately if an arrhythmia occurs. Many patients will have ventricular extrasystoles during exercise. These can be ignored unless their frequency begins to rise.

5. The test should be stopped if the ST segment in any lead becomes depressed by 4 mm.

Horizontal depression of 2 mm in any lead is usually taken as indicating that a diagnosis of ischaemia can be made (a 'positive' test), and if the aim of the test is to confirm or refute a diagnosis of angina there is no point in continuing once this has occurred. It may, however, be useful to find out just how much a patient can do, and if this is the aim of the test it is not unreasonable to continue, if the patient's symptoms are not severe.

Interpretation of ECG changes during exercise testing

The final report of the test should indicate the duration of exercise, the workload achieved, the maximum heart rate and systolic pressure, the reason for discontinuing the test, and a description of any arrhythmias or ST segment changes.

An exercise test is usually considered 'positive' for ischaemia if horizontal or downward-sloping ST segment depression of 2 mm or more develops during exercise, and resolves on resting. By convention, ST segment depression is measured relative to the ECG baseline (between the T and P waves) 60–80 ms after the J point (the point of inflection at the junction of the S wave and the ST segment). A diagnosis of ischaemia becomes almost certain if these changes are accompanied by the appearance and then disappearance of angina. Figs 6.43 and 6.44 show an ECG that was normal when the patient was at rest, but which demonstrated clear ischaemia during exercise. Box 6.8 lists the normal changes in the ECG during exercise, and Box 6.9 lists the changes suggesting a high probability of coronary disease.

When the J point and the ST segment become depressed during exercise, but the ST segment slopes upwards, the change is not an indication of ischaemia (Figs 6.45 and 6.46). Deciding whether ST segment depression slopes upwards or is horizontal can be quite difficult.

In a patient suspected of having coronary disease, exercise testing has a sensitivity of 68% and a specificity of 77%. All tests at times give false positive and false negative results, reflecting their specificity and sensitivity, and false positive tests are particularly common in middle-aged women. In an asymptomatic subject in whom the likelihood of coronary disease is low, the chance of a false positive result may be higher than the chance of a true positive. Also, the greater the likelihood that the patient has coronary disease, the more likely it is

> **BOX 6.8 Normal ECG Changes During Exercise**
>
> - P wave increases in height
> - R wave decreases in height
> - J point becomes depressed
> - ST segment becomes upward-sloping
> - QT interval shortens
> - T wave decreases in height

> **BOX 6.9 Changes on Exercise Suggesting a High Probability of Coronary Artery Disease**
>
> ECG changes
> - Horizontal ST segment depression of > 2 mm
> - Downward-sloping ST segment depression
> - Positive response (i.e. ST segment changes) within 6 min
> - Persistence of ST segment depression for more than 6 min into recovery
> - ST segment depression in five or more leads
>
> Other changes
> - Exertional hypotension

that a positive test is 'true' rather than 'false'. The statistics (Bayes' theorem) may seem complex, but the important thing is to remember that exercise testing is not infallible.

Risks of exercise testing

Exercise testing involves a risk of about 1 in 5000 of the development of ventricular tachycardia or ventricular fibrillation, and a risk of about 1 in 10,000 tests of myocardial infarction or death. There is also a risk of injury if the patient falls, or jumps, off the treadmill. Box 6.10 lists some contraindications of exercise testing.

Fig. 6.43

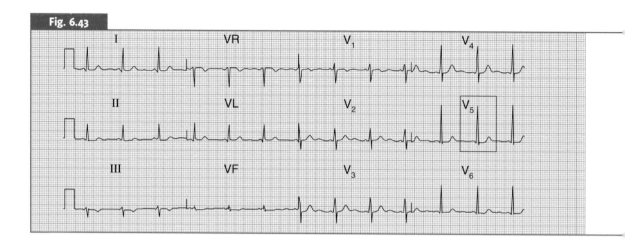

Fig. 6.44

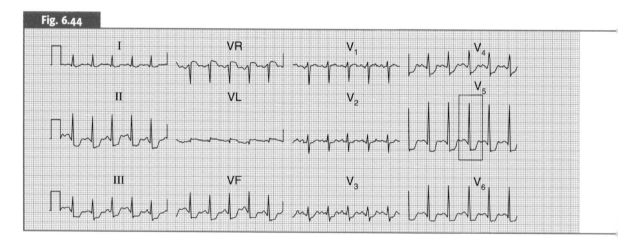

Probably normal record

NOTE

- Sinus rhythm
- Normal axis
- Normal QRS complexes
- Some nonspecific T wave change
  in leads III, VF

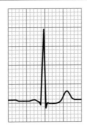

Normal ST segment in lead V_5

Exercise-induced ischaemia

NOTE

- Same patient as in Fig. 6.43
- Sinus rhythm, 138 bpm
- Horizontal ST segment depression in
  leads II–III, VF, V_4–V_6

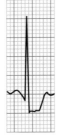

Horizontal ST segment depression in lead V_5

Fig. 6.45

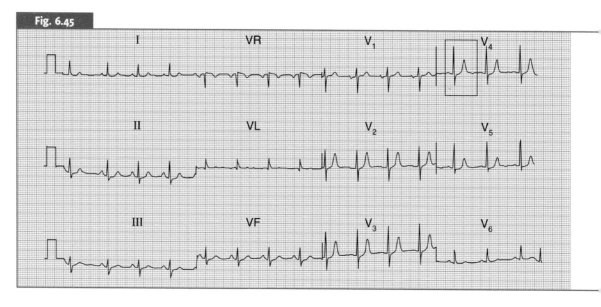

Fig. 6.46

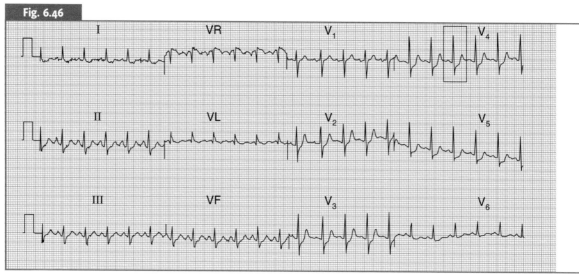

Normal ECG
NOTE

- Sinus rhythm
- Normal axis
- Normal QRS complexes
- Possible minimal ST segment depression in lead V_5

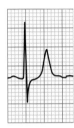

Normal ST segment in lead V_4

BOX 6.10 Contraindications of Exercise Testing

- Acute myocardial infarction within preceding 4–6 days
- Unstable angina
- Uncontrolled heart failure
- Acute myocarditis or pericarditis
- Deep vein thrombosis
- Uncontrolled hypertension (systolic > 220 mmHg, diastolic > 120 mmHg)
- Severe aortic stenosis
- Severe hypertrophic cardiomyopathy
- Untreated life-threatening arrhythmia

Exercise-induced ST segment depression
NOTE

- Same patient as Fig. 6.45
- On exercise there is ST segment depression which slopes upwards
- This is not diagnostic of ischaemia, but the change in lead V_5 is suspicious

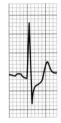

Upward-sloping ST segment depression in lead V_4

Fig. 6.47

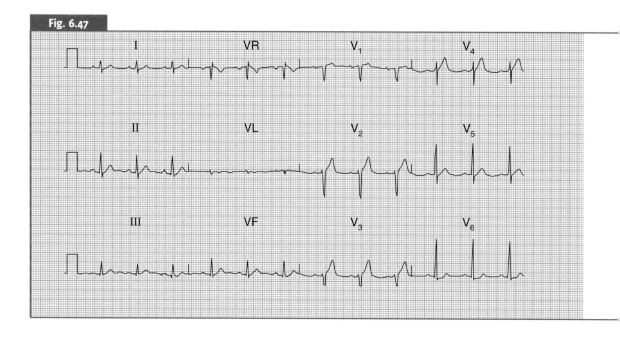

Fig. 6.48

Exercise-induced ventricular extrasystoles

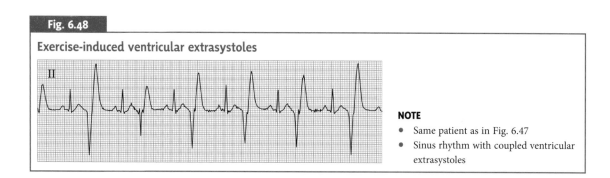

NOTE

- Same patient as in Fig. 6.47
- Sinus rhythm with coupled ventricular extrasystoles

The ECGs in Figs 6.47–6.49 are from a patient whose resting ECG was normal, but as the test proceeded he began to develop ventricular extrasystoles and then suddenly developed ventricular fibrillation. This demonstrates the need for full resuscitation facilities to be available at the time of exercise testing.

Management of chest pain

For detailed discussion of the acute and chronic management of ischaemic or other causes of chest pain, readers are encouraged to refer to contemporary international guidelines.

Pre-exercise: normal ECG

NOTE

- Sinus rhythm
- Heart rate 75 bpm
- Possible nonspecific ST segment depression in lead V_6

| **Fig. 6.49** |

Exercise-induced ventricular fibrillation

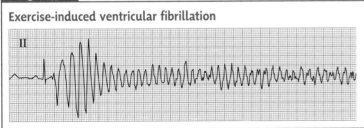

NOTE

- Same patient as in Figs 6.47 and 6.48
- One sinus beat is followed by an extrasystole with the R on T phenomenon
- A few beats of ventricular tachycardia decay into ventricular fibrillation

The ECG in patients with breathlessness

7

History and examination	255
Rhythm problems	257
The ECG in disorders affecting the left side of the heart	259
The ECG in left atrial hypertrophy	259
The ECG in left ventricular hypertrophy	259
ECGs that can mimic left ventricular hypertrophy	265
The ECG in disorders affecting the right side of the heart	269
The ECG in right atrial hypertrophy	269
The ECG in right ventricular hypertrophy	273
What to do	278
Cardiac resynchronization therapy	278

HISTORY AND EXAMINATION

There are many causes of breathlessness (see Box 7.1). Everyone is breathless at times, but people who are physically unfit or who are overweight will be more breathless than others. Breathlessness can also result from anxiety, but when it is due to physical illness the important causes are anaemia, heart disease and lung disease; a combination of causes is common. Apart from ischaemia (see Ch. 6), cardiac diseases causing breathlessness include valve disease, cardiomyopathy and myocarditis. Box 7.2 summarizes the effects of these conditions on the heart, and the corresponding ECG features. The most important function of the history is to help to determine whether the patient does indeed have a physical illness and, if so, which system is affected.

Breathlessness in heart disease is due to either increased lung stiffness, as a result of pulmonary

---

BOX 7.1 Underlying Causes of Breathlessness

Physiological and psychological
- Lack of fitness
- Obesity
- Pregnancy
- Locomotor diseases (including ankylosing spondylitis and neurological diseases)
- Anxiety

Heart disease left ventricular failure
- Ischaemia
- Mitral regurgitation
- Aortic stenosis
- Aortic regurgitation
- Congenital disease
- Cardiomyopathy
- Myocarditis
- Arrhythmias

Heart disease with high left atrial pressure
- Mitral stenosis
- Atrial myxoma

Lung disease
- Chronic obstructive pulmonary disease
- Any interstitial lung disease (e.g. infection, tumour, infiltration)
- Pulmonary embolism
- Pleural effusion
- Pneumothorax

Pericardial disease
- Constrictive pericarditis

Anaemia
- Blood loss

BOX 7.2 The ECG in Valve Disease

Mitral stenosis
- Atrial fibrillation
- Left atrial hypertrophy, if in sinus rhythm
- Right ventricular hypertrophy

Mitral regurgitation
- Atrial fibrillation
- Left atrial hypertrophy, if in sinus rhythm
- Left ventricular hypertrophy

Aortic stenosis
- Left ventricular hypertrophy
- Incomplete left bundle branch block (i.e. loss of Q waves in leads V_5–V_6)
- Left bundle branch block

Aortic regurgitation
- Left ventricular hypertrophy
- Prominent but narrow Q wave in lead V_6
- Left anterior hemiblock
- Occasionally, left bundle branch block

Mitral valve prolapse
- Sinus rhythm, or wide variety of arrhythmias
- Inverted T waves in leads II–III, VF
- T wave inversion in precordial leads
- ST segment depression
- Exercise-induced ventricular arrhythmias

Note: ECG abnormalities are highly variable between individuals and, although suggestive, no pattern of findings can be considered diagnostic without corroborative clinical and imaging findings

congestion, or pulmonary oedema. Pulmonary congestion occurs when the left atrial pressure is high. A high left atrial pressure occurs either in mitral stenosis or in left ventricular failure. Pulmonary oedema occurs when the left atrial pressure exceeds the oncotic pressure exerted by the plasma proteins.

Congestive cardiac failure (right heart failure secondary to left heart failure) can be difficult to distinguish from cor pulmonale (right heart failure due to lung disease). With both, the patient is breathless. Both are associated with pulmonary crackles in left heart failure due to pulmonary oedema, and in cor pulmonale due to the lung disease. Also in both, the patient may complain of orthopnoea. Both pulmonary congestion and lung disease can cause a diffuse wheeze. The diagnosis therefore depends on a positive identification, either in the history, examination or investigations, of heart or lung disease.

The main value of the ECG in patients with breathlessness is to indicate whether heart disease of any sort is present, and to some extent whether the left or the right side of the heart is affected. The ECG is best at identifying rhythm abnormalities (which may lead to left ventricular impairment and so to breathlessness) and conditions affecting the left ventricle, particularly ischaemia. A patient with a completely normal ECG is unlikely to have left ventricular failure, although of course there are exceptions. Lung disease eventually affects the right side of the heart and may cause ECG changes, suggesting that significant lung disease is present.

RHYTHM PROBLEMS

A sudden rhythm change is a common cause of breathlessness, and even of frank pulmonary oedema. Arrhythmias can be paroxysmal, so the patient may be in sinus rhythm when examined, and a patient who is suddenly breathless may not be aware of an arrhythmia. When sudden breathlessness is associated with palpitations it is important to establish whether the breathlessness or the palpitations came first; palpitations following breathlessness may be due to the sinus tachycardia of anxiety. The ECG in Fig. 7.1 is from a patient who developed pulmonary oedema due to the onset of uncontrolled atrial fibrillation.

Less dramatic rhythm abnormalities can also contribute to breathlessness, especially to breathlessness on exertion. This is true of both fast and slow rhythms. The ECG in Fig. 7.2 is from a patient who had atrial fibrillation but who was breathless on exercise partly because of ventricular bigeminy (a coupled ventricular extrasystole following each normally conducted QRS complex), which markedly reduced cardiac output as a result of an effective halving of the heart rate.

Fig. 7.1

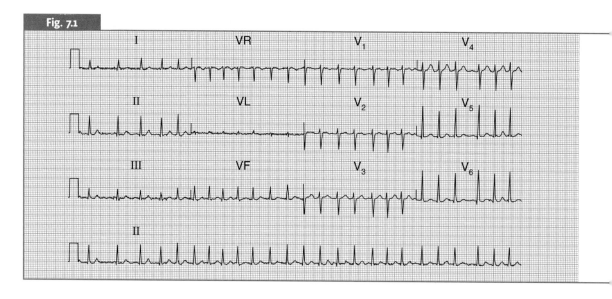

Fig. 7.2

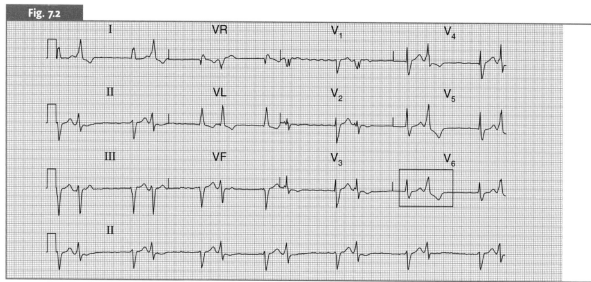

Uncontrolled atrial fibrillation

NOTE

- Atrial fibrillation, with ventricular rate 170 bpm
- No other abnormalities
- No evidence of digoxin effect

Atrial fibrillation with coupled ventricular extrasystoles

NOTE

- Atrial fibrillation, with slow and regular ventricular response
- Coupled ventricular extrasystoles
- In supraventricular beats, leads V_5–V_6 show a deep wide S wave, suggesting right bundle branch block
- Digoxin toxicity

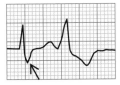

Deep wide S wave in supraventricular beat in lead V_6

THE ECG IN DISORDERS AFFECTING THE LEFT SIDE OF THE HEART

The ECG in left atrial hypertrophy

Left atrial hypertrophy causes a double (bifid) P wave. Left atrial hypertrophy without left ventricular hypertrophy is classically due to mitral stenosis, so the bifid P wave is sometimes called 'P mitrale'. This is misleading, because most patients whose ECGs have bifid P waves either have left ventricular hypertrophy that is not obvious on the ECG or, and perhaps this is more common, have a perfectly normal heart (see Ch. 1, p. 14; Fig. 1.13). The bifid P wave is thus not a useful measure of left atrial hypertrophy.

Fig. 7.3 shows an ECG with a bifid P wave indicating left atrial hypertrophy. This was confirmed by echocardiography in the patient, who also had concentric left ventricular hypertrophy due to hypertension.

Significant mitral stenosis usually, but not always, leads to atrial fibrillation, in which no P waves, bifid or otherwise, can be seen. Occasional patients, such as the one whose ECG is shown in Fig. 7.4, develop pulmonary hypertension and remain in sinus rhythm. There is then a combination of a bifid P wave with evidence of right ventricular hypertrophy. This combination does suggest a diagnosis of severe mitral stenosis.

The ECG in left ventricular hypertrophy

Left ventricular hypertrophy may be caused by hypertension, aortic stenosis or incompetence, or mitral incompetence.

The ECG features of left ventricular hypertrophy are:
- an increased height of the QRS complex (although this may be normal – see Ch. 1, pp. 24-26 and ECGs 1.24 and 1.25)
- inverted T waves in the leads that 'look at' the left ventricle I, VL and V_5–V_6.

Left axis deviation is not uncommon, but is due more to fibrosis causing left anterior hemiblock than to the left ventricular hypertrophy itself.

Fig. 7.3

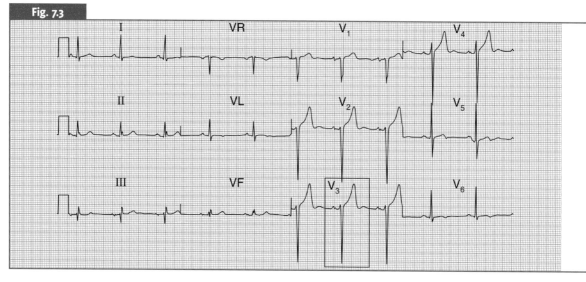

Fig. 7.4

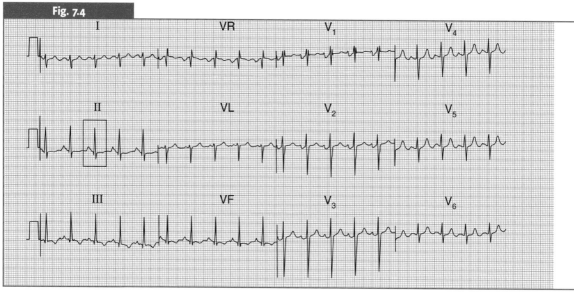

Left atrial hypertrophy and left ventricular hypertrophy

NOTE

- Sinus rhythm
- Bifid P waves
- Normal axis
- Tall QRS complexes
- Inverted T waves in lead V_6, suggesting left ventricular hypertrophy

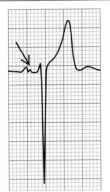

Bifid P wave in lead V_3

Mitral stenosis and pulmonary hypertension

NOTE

- Sinus rhythm
- Bifid P wave (best seen in lead II)
- Right axis deviation
- Partial right bundle branch block pattern
- Persistent S wave in lead V_6

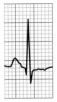

Bifid P wave in lead II

The complete ECG picture of left ventricular hypertrophy is easy to recognize. The ECG in Fig. 7.5 is from a patient with severe and untreated hypertension. It shows the 'voltage criteria' which, when combined with the T wave inversion in the lateral leads, probably are significant. In this case, the small Q waves in the lateral leads are septal and do not indicate a previous infarction. Note that the T wave inversion is most prominent in lead V_6, and becomes progressively less so in leads V_5 and V_4. This pattern of T wave inversion is sometimes referred to as 'left ventricular strain', but this is an old-fashioned and essentially meaningless term.

The most important cause of severe left ventricular hypertrophy is aortic valve disease: when aortic stenosis or incompetence causes left ventricular hypertrophy, aortic valve replacement must be considered. Aortic valve disease is frequently associated with left bundle branch block (LBBB) (Fig. 7.6), which completely masks any evidence of left ventricular hypertrophy. The patient who is

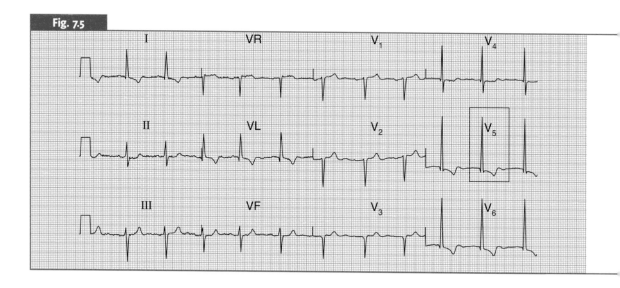

Fig. 7.5

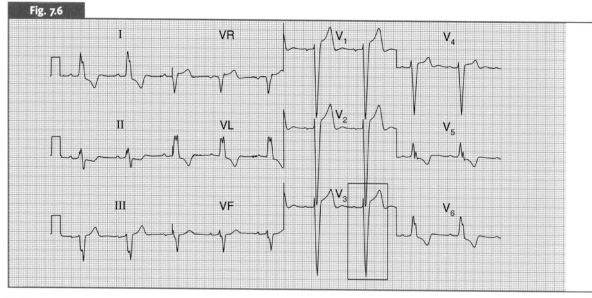

Fig. 7.6

Left ventricular hypertrophy
NOTE
- Sinus rhythm
- Voltage criteria for left ventricular hypertrophy
- Inverted T waves in leads I, VL, V_5–V_6

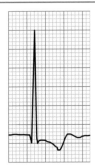

Tall R wave and inverted T wave in lead V_5

Left bundle branch block with aortic stenosis
NOTE
- Sinus rhythm
- Normal axis
- Broad QRS complexes with LBBB pattern
- Very deep S waves in lead V_3
- Inverted T waves in leads I, VL, V_5–V_6

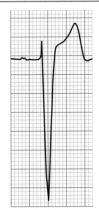

Broad QRS complex and deep S wave in lead V_3

Fig. 7.7

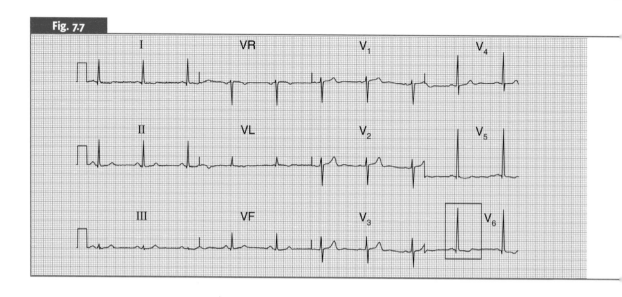

Fig. 7.8

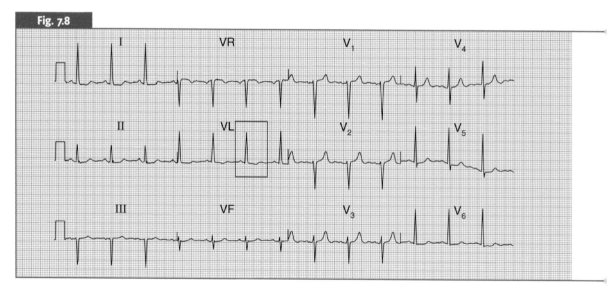

Left ventricular hypertrophy
NOTE

- Sinus rhythm
- Normal axis
- Voltage criteria for left ventricular hypertrophy not met
- Inverted T waves in leads I, VL, V_6

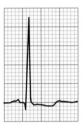

Normal R wave and inverted T wave in lead V_6

Left ventricular hypertrophy with severe aortic stenosis
NOTE

- Sinus rhythm
- Normal axis
- Voltage criteria for left ventricular hypertrophy not met
- Minor ST segment/T wave changes in leads I, VL, V_6

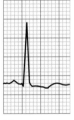

Minor ST segment/T wave changes in lead VL

breathless, or who has chest pain or dizziness, and has signs of aortic valve disease and an ECG showing LBBB, needs urgent investigation. However, it is important to remember the ECG cannot be used to assess severity or monitor progression of valvular heart disease. This will usually be assessed by echocardiography.

Unfortunately, therefore, the severity of ECG changes correlates poorly with the severity of left ventricular hypertrophy and is an unreliable guide to the importance of the underlying cardiac problem. The ECG in Fig. 7.7 shows lateral T wave inversion, but does not meet the 'voltage criteria', in a patient with moderate aortic stenosis (aortic valve gradient 60 mmHg).

In contrast, the ECG in Fig. 7.8 is from a patient with severe aortic stenosis and an aortic valve gradient of > 120 mmHg, yet it shows little to suggest severe ventricular hypertrophy.

ECGs that can mimic left ventricular hypertrophy

The problems of differentiating between lateral T wave changes due to left ventricular hypertrophy and those due to ischaemia have been discussed in Chapter 6, p. 241. The history and physical examination become extremely important, and the ECG must not be viewed in isolation and further investigations may be merited. The ECG in Fig. 7.9 is from a patient with chest pain that was compatible with, but not diagnostic of, angina and who had physical signs suggesting mild aortic stenosis. The T wave inversion is more prominent in leads V_4 and V_5 than in V_6, and is present in V_3. The T waves are upright in leads I and VL. These changes point to ischaemia rather than left ventricular hypertrophy, and ischaemia proved to be present in this patient.

The ECG in Fig. 7.10 is from a patient with hypertension and breathlessness. He was shown to have left ventricular hypertrophy and coronary disease, but all the changes here could have been due to left ventricular hypertrophy alone.

Fig. 7.9

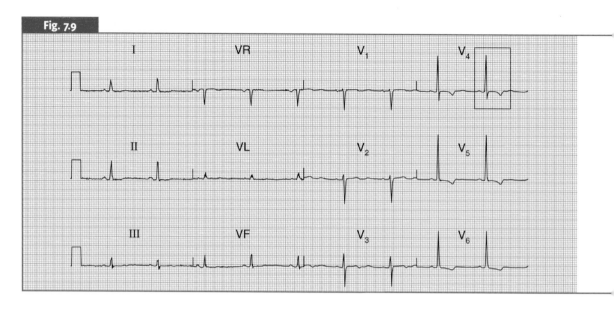

Fig. 7.10

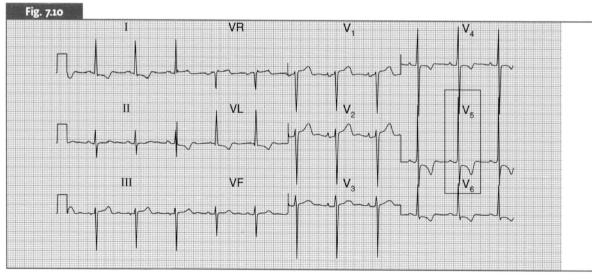

Probable ischaemia

NOTE

- Sinus rhythm
- Normal axis
- T wave inversion in leads II and V_3–V_6, but most prominent in V_4–V_5

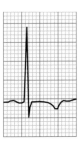

Inverted T wave in lead V_4

When a breathless patient has an ECG with gross lateral T wave changes (Fig. 7.11), hypertrophic cardiomyopathy is a possibility.

Lateral T wave changes associated with left anterior hemiblock often accompany left ventricular hypertrophy. However, there was no echocardiographic evidence of this in the patient whose ECG is shown in Fig. 7.12. Here the changes must be due to conducting system disease.

Another example of a conducting tissue abnormality that could be mistaken for left ventricular hypertrophy is the Wolff–Parkinson–White (WPW) syndrome. The ECG in Fig. 7.13 is from a young man with WPW syndrome type B. There is left ventricular hypertrophy according to voltage criteria, and there is also lateral T wave inversion, but the diagnosis is made from the short PR intervals and the delta waves. The height of the QRS complexes and the T wave inversion in this situation do not indicate left ventricular hypertrophy.

Left ventricular hypertrophy, ischaemia

NOTE

- Sinus rhythm
- Bifid P waves, best seen in lead I
- Normal axis
- T wave inversion in leads I, VL and V_3–V_6, but most prominent in V_5

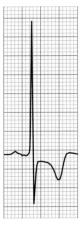

Maximal T wave inversion in lead V_5

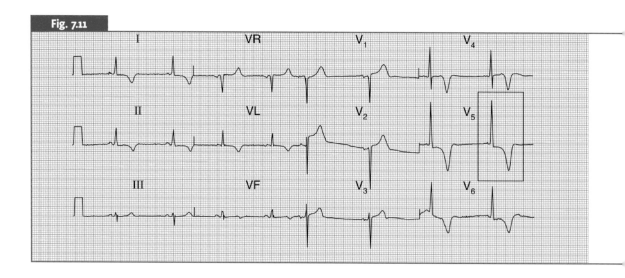

Fig. 7.11

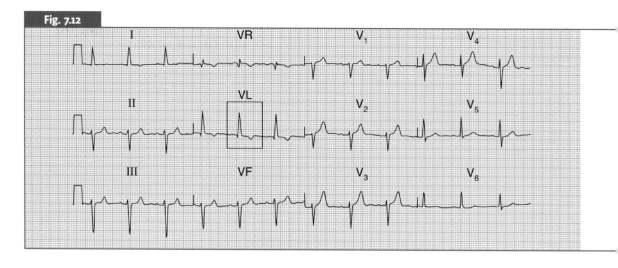

Fig. 7.12

Hypertrophic cardiomyopathy
NOTE
- Sinus rhythm
- Bifid P wave, best seen in lead V_4
- Voltage criteria for left ventricular hypertrophy not met
- Gross T wave inversion in leads V_4–V_6

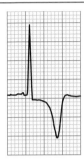

Normal R wave and dramatic T wave inversion in lead V_5

Left anterior hemiblock
NOTE
- Sinus rhythm
- Left axis deviation
- Inverted T waves in leads I, VL

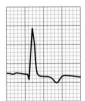

Inverted T wave in lead VL

THE ECG IN DISORDERS AFFECTING THE RIGHT SIDE OF THE HEART

Right-sided heart disease can be the result of chronic lung disease (e.g. chronic obstructive airways disease, bronchiectasis), pulmonary embolism (especially when repeated episodes cause thromboembolic pulmonary hypertension; see also Ch. 6, p. 231), idiopathic pulmonary hypertension, or congenital heart disease. Any of these can cause right ventricular hypertrophy, but none of them causes a specific ECG abnormality (Boxes 7.3 and 7.4).

The ECG in right atrial hypertrophy

Right atrial hypertrophy causes tall and peaked P waves, which are sometimes described as 'P pulmonale'. There is, in fact, such variation within the normal range of P waves that the diagnosis of right atrial hypertrophy is difficult to make. Its presence can be inferred when peaked P waves are associated with the ECG changes of right ventricular

Fig. 7.13

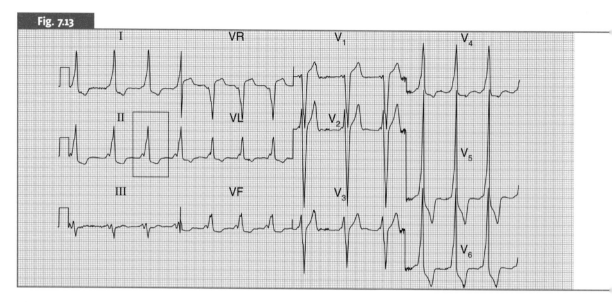

Fig. 7.14

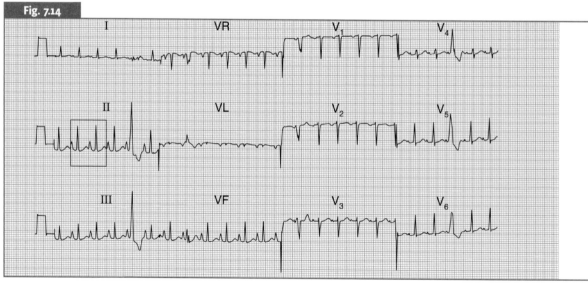

The Wolff–Parkinson–White syndrome (no left ventricular hypertrophy)

NOTE

- Short PR interval
- Broad QRS complexes with delta waves
- Very tall R waves
- Inverted T waves in leads I, II, VL, V_4–V_6

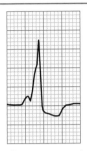

Short PR interval and delta wave in lead II

Right atrial hypertrophy

NOTE

- Sinus rhythm with occasional aberrant conduction
- Tall and peaked P waves
- No other abnormality
- In this case the right atrial hypertrophy was due to tricuspid stenosis

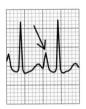

Peaked P wave in lead II

BOX 7.3 The ECG in Pulmonary Embolism

- Sinus tachycardia
- Atrial arrhythmias
- Right atrial hypertrophy
- Right ventricular hypertrophy
- Right axis deviation
- Clockwise rotation, with persistent S wave in lead V_6
- Right bundle branch block
- Combination of S wave in lead I with Q wave and inverted T wave in lead III

hypertrophy. Evidence of right atrial hypertrophy without right ventricular hypertrophy will usually only be seen in rare patients with isolated tricuspid stenosis (Fig. 7.14).

The ECG in Fig. 7.15 is from a patient with right atrial and right ventricular hypertrophy due to severe chronic obstructive pulmonary disease.

271

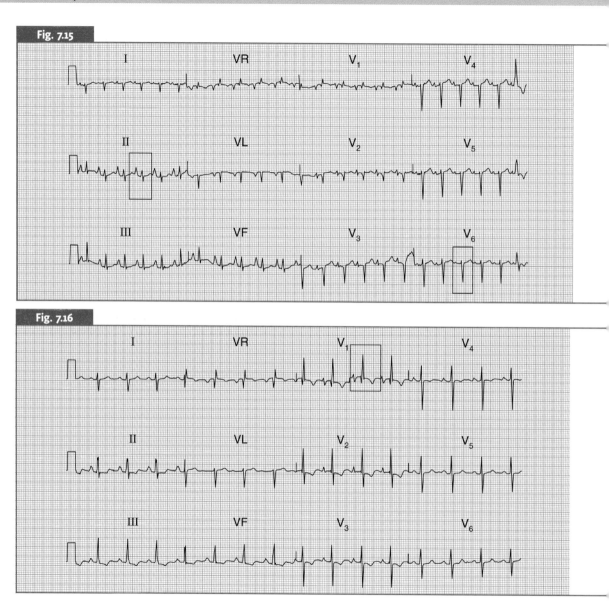

Fig. 7.15

Fig. 7.16

Right atrial and right ventricular hypertrophy

NOTE

- Peaked P waves, especially in lead II
- Right axis deviation
- Persistent S waves in lead V_6 (clockwise rotation) suggest chronic lung disease

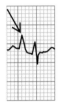 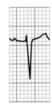

Peaked P wave in lead II   Persistent S wave in lead V_6

Marked right ventricular hypertrophy

NOTE

- Sinus rhythm
- Peaked P waves
- Right axis deviation
- Dominant R waves in lead V_1
- Persistent S waves in lead V_6

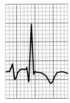

Dominant R wave in lead V_1

BOX 7.4 The ECG in Chronic Obstructive Pulmonary Disease

- Small QRS complexes
- Right atrial hypertrophy (P pulmonale)
- Right axis deviation
- Right ventricular hypertrophy
- Clockwise rotation, with persistent, deep S wave in lead V_6
- Right bundle branch block

The ECG in right ventricular hypertrophy

The ECG changes associated with right ventricular hypertrophy are:

- right axis deviation
- a dominant R wave in lead V_1
- clockwise rotation of the heart: as the septum is displaced laterally, the transition of the QRS complex in the chest leads from a right to a left ventricular configuration occurs in leads V_4–V_6 instead of V_2–V_4; there is thus a persistent S wave in lead V_6, which normally does not show an S wave at all
- inversion of the T wave in leads that 'look at' the right ventricle: Vi, V_2 and occasionally V_3.

In extreme cases it is easy to diagnose right ventricular hypertrophy from the ECG. The ECG in Fig. 7.16 came from a patient incapacitated by breathlessness due to primary pulmonary hypertension.

As with the ECG in left ventricular hypertrophy, none of the ECG changes of right ventricular hypertrophy individually provide unequivocal evidence of right ventricular hypertrophy (Table 7.1). Conversely, it is possible to have marked right ventricular hypertrophy without all the typical ECG features being present. Minor degrees of right axis deviation are seen in normal people, and a dominant R wave in lead V_1 is occasionally seen in normal people, although it is never more than 3 or 4 mm tall. A dominant

Fig. 7.17

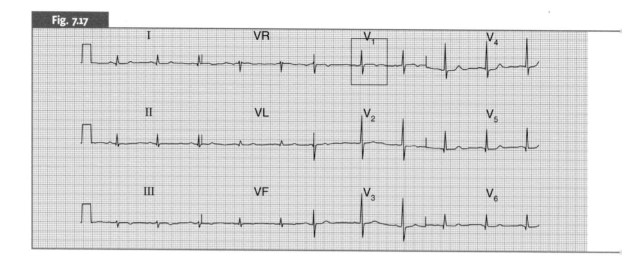

Fig. 7.18

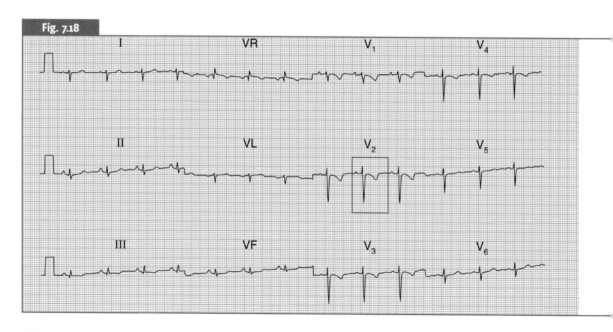

Probable normal variant

NOTE

- Sinus rhythm
- Normal axis
- Dominant R waves in lead V_1
- Inverted T waves in lead III

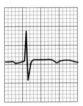

Dominant R wave in lead V_1

Right ventricular hypertrophy

NOTE

- Sinus rhythm
- Right axis deviation
- No dominant R waves in lead V_1
- Inverted T waves in leads V_1–V_4, maximal in lead V_1
- Persistent S waves in lead V_6

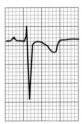

Inverted T wave in lead V_2

TABLE 7.1 Possible Alternative Causes of the ECG Appearance of Right Ventricular Hypertrophy

ECG feature	Cause
Right axis deviation	Normal in tall thin people
Dominant R wave in lead V_1	Normal variant
	Posterior infarction The Wolff–Parkinson–White syndrome Right bundle branch block of any cause
Inverted T waves in leads V_1–V_2	Normal variant, especially in black people
	Anterior non-ST segment elevation acute coronary syndrome The Wolff–Parkinson–White syndrome Right bundle branch block of any cause Cardiomyopathy
Apparent clockwise rotation	Dextrocardia

R wave in lead V_1 may also indicate a 'true posterior' myocardial infarction (see Ch. 6, p. 237). There may be variation in the T wave inversion in leads V_1 and V_2 in normal subjects (see Ch. 1, p. 41, Figs 1.41 and 1.42) and, particularly in black people, the T wave can be inverted in leads V_2 and V_3.

The ECG in Fig. 7.17 shows a dominant R wave in lead V_1 but no other evidence of right ventricular hypertrophy. This could indicate a posterior myocardial infarction (see Ch. 6, p. 236), but this trace was from a young man who was asymptomatic, who had no abnormalities on examination, and whose echocardiogram was normal. This is a normal variant.

The ECG in Fig. 7.18 is from a young woman who had become progressively more breathless since the birth of

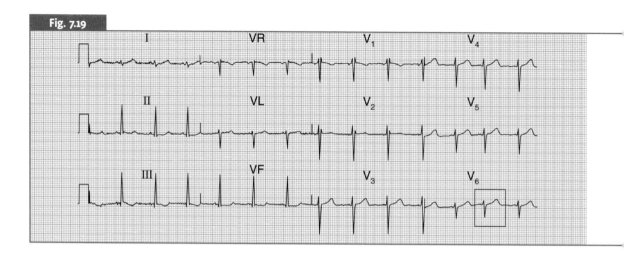

Fig. 7.19

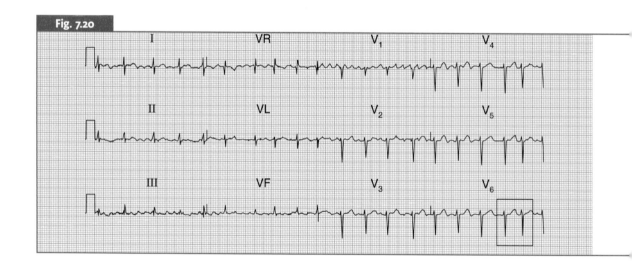

Fig. 7.20

Chronic lung disease

NOTE

- Sinus rhythm
- Right axis deviation
- Prominent S waves in lead V$_6$
- Nonspecific T wave changes in leads III and VF

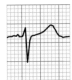

Persistent S wave in lead V$_6$

Pulmonary embolus

NOTE

- Atrial fibrillation, ventricular rate 114 bpm
- Dominant S wave in lead V$_6$
- No other evidence of right ventricular hypertrophy

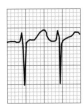

Persistent S wave in lead V$_6$

her baby 4 months previously. She had had no chest pain. No previous ECGs were available. The anterior T wave changes could be a normal variant in a black woman. T wave inversion in leads V$_3$–V$_4$ could indicate anterior ischaemia, but the important point here is that the T wave inversion is most prominent in leads Vi–V$_2$, and becomes progressively less in V$_3$–V$_4$. This is characteristic of T wave inversion due to right ventricular hypertrophy. In this case the T wave inversion, combined with right axis deviation and a persistent S wave in lead V$_6$, suggests right ventricular hypertrophy. The patient was shown to have had recurrent small pulmonary emboli.

A prominent S wave in lead V$_6$ is sometimes called 'persistent' because this lead should show a pure left ventricular type of complex with a dominant R wave and no S wave. The 'transition point', when the R and S waves are equal, indicates the position of the interventricular septum and this is normally under the position of lead V$_3$ or V$_4$. In the ECG in Fig. 7.19, a transition point is not present at all, and lead V$_6$ shows a small R wave and a dominant S wave. This is due to the right ventricle underlying more of the precordium than usual. This change is characteristic of chronic lung disease.

When breathlessness is accompanied by a sudden change in rotation, a pulmonary embolus is likely. The ECG in Fig. 7.20 is from a patient who had had a normal preoperative ECG but who developed breathlessness with atrial fibrillation a week after cholecystectomy. The deep S wave in lead V$_6$ is the pointer towards a pulmonary embolus being the cause of the atrial fibrillation.

As with the ECG in left ventricular hypertrophy, it is the appearance of changes in serial recordings that provides the best evidence of minor or moderate degrees of right ventricular hypertrophy. In the majority of cases in which the ECG suggests right ventricular hypertrophy, it is not possible to diagnose the underlying disease process with certainty.

WHAT TO DO

In most patients with breathlessness, the ECG does not contribute very much to diagnosis and management, and the important thing is to treat the patient and not the ECG.

The ECG cannot diagnose heart failure, although heart failure is unlikely if the ECG is totally normal. By demonstrating ischaemia or enlargement of one or more of the cardiac chambers, the ECG may help to identify the underlying disease that requires treatment. However, the symptoms of acute heart failure need empirical treatment whatever the ECG shows, and this should not be delayed while an ECG is being recorded.

The ECG can provide confirmatory evidence that breathlessness is due to a pulmonary embolus or chronic lung disease, but it is an unreliable way of making this diagnosis and treatment cannot depend on the ECG. Similarly, the ECG will not help in the diagnosis of anaemia, although it may show ischaemic changes.

In general then, the management of the breathless patient does not depend on the ECG unless breathlessness is due to heart failure which is secondary to an arrhythmia. In such cases, the ECG is essential both for diagnosis and for monitoring the response to therapy.

Cardiac resynchronization therapy

Patients with severe heart failure, especially those whose ECG shows LBBB with a broad QRS complex, may have dyssynchronous cardiac contraction. Instead of both sides of the left ventricle contracting simultaneously in systole, there is a substantial delay between contraction of the left ventricular septum and the free wall. This reduces the stroke volume and exacerbates the heart failure. Contraction can be resynchronized by pacing the left ventricular free wall and the septum simultaneously. This is achieved by two pacing leads – one placed in a branch of the coronary sinus (the venous side of the coronary circulation, which drains into the right atrium), with a second, right ventricular lead to pace the septum. This technique, cardiac resynchronization therapy (CRT), is also known as biventricular pacing, or simply 'bivent'. Resynchronization improves both cardiac output and symptomatic heart failure. In addition to right ventricular and coronary sinus leads, there will usually be an atrial lead if sinus rhythm is present, because atrial systole may make an important contribution to cardiac output (Fig. 7.21). Devices aimed at pacing the His conducting tissue are also in use in some centres (see Ch. 5, Figs 5.30, 5.31 and 5.32). These devices encourage a more physiological cardiac depolarization by exploiting the native conducting system.

Indications for CRT

Numerous clinical studies have shown that in appropriate patients CRT can improve left ventricular function and ejection fraction, and can improve exercise capacity. In patients still symptomatic from heart failure despite optimal medical therapy, CRT has been shown to reduce morbidity and all-cause mortality. CRT is therefore now considered a standard therapy; its indications are listed in Box 7.5. Since it is an invasive and costly procedure, patient selection is clearly extremely important with implantation according to American Heart Association/European Society of Cardiology guidelines.

ECG appearance

Biventricular pacing needs to be continuous, or 'obligate' (as opposed to 'on demand'), because resynchronization cannot be achieved unless the heart is in a paced rhythm. If necessary, pacing is ensured by careful programming

Fig. 7.21

Cardiac resynchronisation pacemaker (CRT)

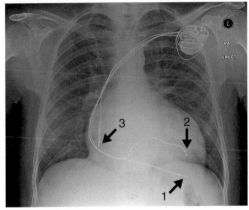
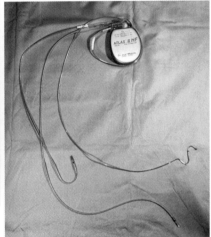

NOTE

- CRT pacemaker prior to implantation (right) and chest X-ray showing implantation position (left)
- Ventricular lead in right ventricular apex position (arrow 1)
- Coronary sinus lead for left ventricular pacing (arrow 2)
- Atrial lead in right atrial appendage position (arrow 3)

BOX 7.5 Indications for Cardiac Resynchronization Therapy

These are continuing to evolve as indications broaden and device costs fall. It is currently recommended for patients:

- on optimal pharmacotherapy
- with an ejection fraction of less than 35%
- with left bundle branch block with a QRS complex longer than 150 ms (or 120–149 ms and with LBBB)
- with heart failure symptoms

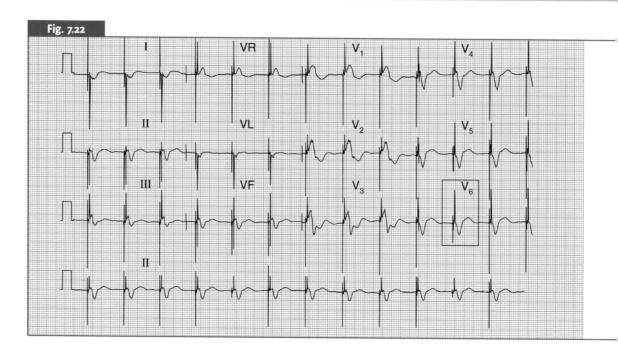

Fig. 7.22

Biventricular pacing

NOTE

- Complex ventricular pacing spike, sometimes with two distinct elements derived from the right ventricular and coronary sinus leads
- Right bundle branch block morphology in the QRS complexes
- Obligate pacing throughout

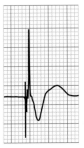

Two juxtaposed pacing spikes

---

of the atrioventricular (AV) delay or by pharmacological suppression of the intrinsic rhythm.

The pacing spike may be complex and may have two components. The QRS complex of the paced beat may have either a narrowed LBBB morphology or a right bundle branch block morphology (Fig. 7.22).

Patients without an atrial lead will usually have atrial fibrillation or atrial flutter.

Specialist functions

Patients with severe left ventricular dysfunction are at increased risk of ventricular arrhythmias, so some CRT devices incorporate a ventricular implanted cardioverter defibrillation element (CRTD). This device will function in the same way as a conventional biventricular pacing device, but with the additional function of an implantable cardioverter defibrillator (ICD) (see Ch. 4, p. 143).

The effects of other conditions on the ECG

8

Artefacts in ECG recordings	**283**
The effects of abnormal muscle movement	283
Hypothermia	283
The ECG in congenital heart disease	**285**
The ECG in systemic diseases	**293**
Thyroid disease	293
Malignancy	295
The effects of serum electrolyte abnormalities on the ECG	**295**
Potassium	295
Magnesium	301
Calcium	301
The effects of medication on the ECG	**301**
Digoxin	301
Other causes of an abnormal ECG	**305**
Trauma	305
Metabolic diseases	305
Cerebrovascular accidents	305
Muscle disease	307

The ECG is not a good method for investigating or diagnosing any condition that is not primarily cardiac. However, some generalized diseases do affect the ECG: it is important to recognize this, and not assume that a patient has heart disease simply because their ECG seems abnormal.

ARTEFACTS IN ECG RECORDINGS

The effects of abnormal muscle movement

Although ECG recorders are designed to be especially sensitive to the electrical frequencies of cardiac muscle contraction, the ECG will also record the contraction of skeletal muscles. The most common pattern of 'ECG abnormality' is a high-frequency oscillation due to general muscular tension in a patient who is not properly relaxed.

Sustained involuntary tremors, such as those associated with Parkinsonism (Fig. 8.1) cause rhythmic ECG abnormalities that may be confused with cardiac arrhythmias.

Hypothermia

Hypothermia causes shivering, and therefore artefacts due to muscular activity. However, there can be other changes in the ECG, and the characteristic ECG feature of hypothermia is the 'J' wave. This is a small hump seen at the end of the QRS complex (Fig. 8.2).

Fig. 8.1

Parkinsonism

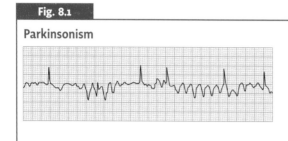

NOTE

- Muscle tremor at 5/s gives an appearance resembling atrial flutter
- The irregular QRS complexes may indicate that the rhythm is actually atrial fibrillation
- This record demonstrates the importance of looking at the patient as well as the ECG

Fig. 8.2

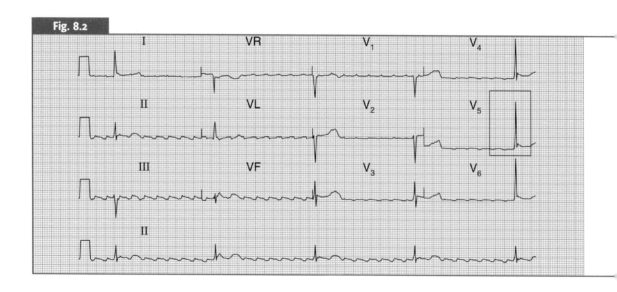

The ECG in Fig. 8.2 was recorded from a 76-year-old woman who was admitted to hospital with a temperature of 30°C after lying for a prolonged period in a freezing house, after a fall. She initially had a heart rate of 26 bpm, and the rhythm was atrial flutter. J waves can be seen in the lateral chest leads. On re-warming, she began to shiver, and, despite the muscle artefact, her heart can be seen to have reverted to sinus rhythm with first degree block. J waves are still visible (Fig. 8.3). When her temperature had returned to normal, the PR interval normalized, and the J waves disappeared (Fig. 8.4).

THE ECG IN CONGENITAL HEART DISEASE

The ECG provides a limited amount of help in the diagnosis of congenital heart disease by showing which chambers of the heart are enlarged. It is important to remember

(see Ch. 1, p. 52) that at birth the ECG of a normal infant shows a pattern of 'right ventricular hypertrophy', and this gradually disappears during the first 2 years of life.

If the infant pattern persists beyond the age of 2 years, right ventricular hypertrophy is indeed present. If there is a left ventricular, or normal adult, pattern before this age, then left ventricular hypertrophy is probably present. In older children, the criteria for left and right ventricular hypertrophy are the same as in adults.

Box 8.1 lists some common congenital disorders and the associated ECG appearances.

Atrial flutter, hypothermia

NOTE

- Atrial flutter with ventricular rate 26 bpm
- J waves visible in leads V_4–V_6

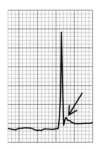

J wave in lead V_5

BOX 8.1 ECG Appearance in Common Congenital Disorders

Right ventricular hypertrophy
- Pulmonary hypertension of any cause (e.g. Eisenmenger's syndrome)
- Severe pulmonary stenosis
- Fallot's tetralogy
- Transposition of the great arteries

Left ventricular hypertrophy
- Aortic stenosis
- Coarctation of the aorta
- Mitral regurgitation
- Obstructive cardiomyopathy

Biventricular hypertrophy
- Ventricular septal defect

Right atrial hypertrophy
- Tricuspid stenosis

Right bundle branch block
- Atrial septal defect
- Complex defects

Left axis deviation
- Endocardial cushion defects
- Corrected transposition

Fig. 8.3

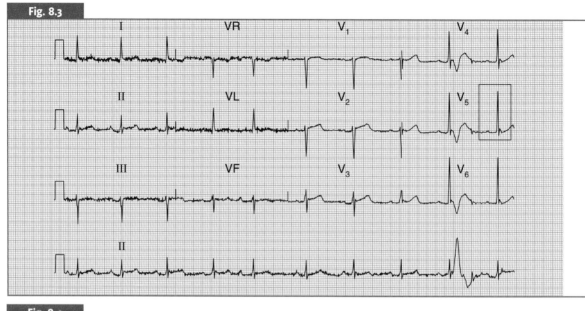

Fig. 8.4

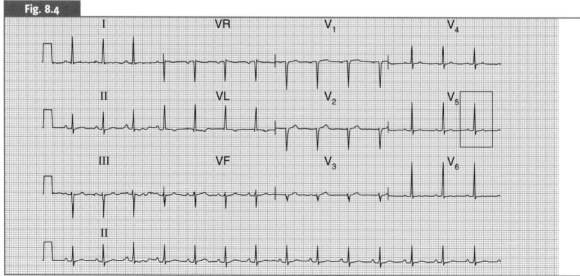

Hypothermia
NOTE
- Same patient as in Figs 8.2 and 8.4
- Sinus rhythm is restored
- The patient has begun to shiver (muscle artefact in the limb leads, with a further artefact in the penultimate complex of the rhythm strip)
- First degree block
- J waves still visible

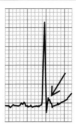

J wave in lead V$_5$

Re-warming after hypothermia
NOTE
- Same patient as in Figs 8.2 and 8.3
- The patient is now in sinus rhythm with a normal PR interval
- J waves have disappeared
- There are some nonspecific ST-segment and T-wave changes in leads I–II, VL, V$_6$

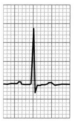

No J wave in lead V$_5$

Fig. 8.5

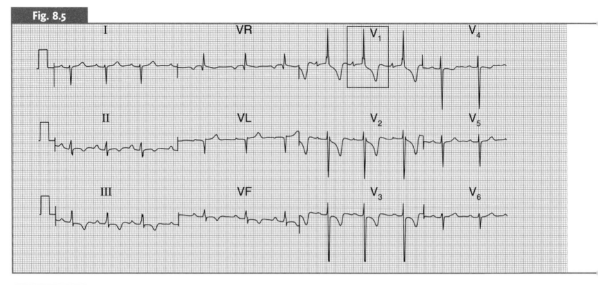

Fig. 8.6

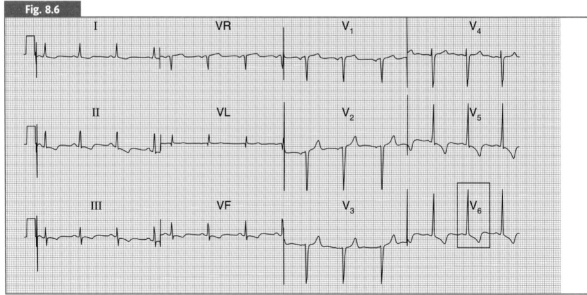

Pulmonary stenosis

NOTE

- Sinus rhythm
- Right axis deviation
- Dominant R waves in lead V_1
- Persistent S waves in lead V_6
- Inverted T waves in leads V_1–V_4

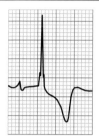

Dominant R wave in lead V_1

Left ventricular hypertrophy

NOTE

- Sinus rhythm
- Normal axis
- Left ventricular hypertrophy according to voltage criteria
- T-wave inversion in leads I, V_5–V_6

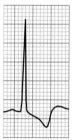

Tall R wave and inverted T wave in lead V_6

The ECG in Fig. 8.5 shows all the features of severe right ventricular hypertrophy: it came from a boy with severe pulmonary stenosis.

The ECG in Fig. 8.6 shows left ventricular hypertrophy, and was recorded in an 8-year-old with severe aortic stenosis.

Fig. 8.7

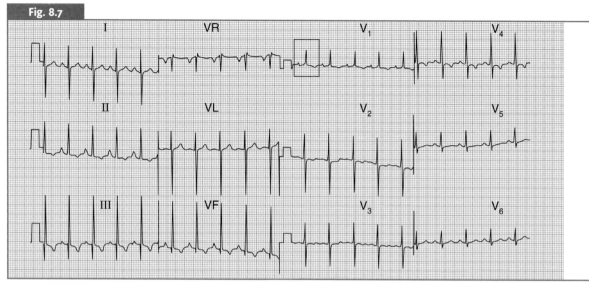

Fig. 8.8

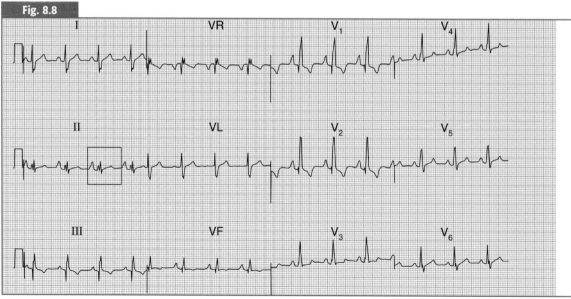

The ECG in Fig. 8.7 shows right ventricular hypertrophy, and came from a young woman who had had a partial correction of Fallot's tetralogy 20 years previously.

The ECG in Fig. 8.8 suggests right atrial hypertrophy and shows right bundle branch block (RBBB). It came from a teenager with Ebstein's anomaly and an atrial septal defect.

It is usually fairly obvious that a patient has congenital heart disease of some sort, but the condition that may be missed is an atrial septal defect. The ECG in Fig. 8.9 is from a 50-year-old woman who complained of mild but increasing breathlessness. She had a rather nonspecific systolic murmur at the left sternal edge. Her GP recorded an ECG which showed RBBB and as a result she had an echocardiogram which showed an atrial septal defect.

Right ventricular hypertrophy in Fallot's tetralogy

NOTE

- Leads V_1–V_6 recorded at half sensitivity
- Sinus rhythm
- Right axis deviation
- Dominant R waves in lead V_1
- T-wave inversion in leads II–III, VF, V_1–V_4

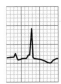

Dominant R wave in lead V_1

Right atrial hypertrophy and right bundle branch block, in Ebstein's anomaly

NOTE

- Sinus rhythm
- Peaked P waves in lead II
- Broad QRS complexes with RBBB pattern

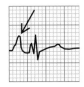

Peaked P wave in lead II

Fig. 8.9

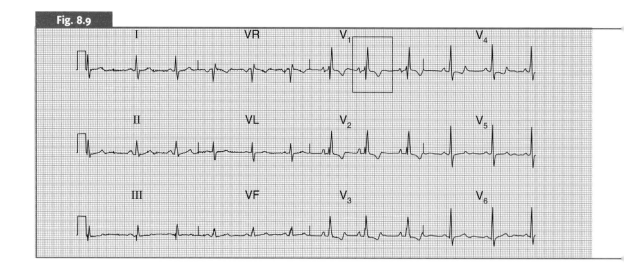

Fig. 8.10

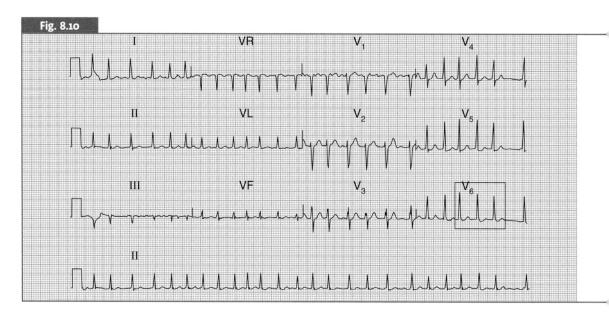

Right bundle branch block with atrial septal defect

NOTE

- Sinus rhythm
- Normal axis
- QRS complex duration within normal limits (108 ms)
- RBBB pattern

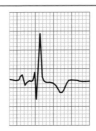

RBBB pattern in lead V_1

Thyrotoxicosis

NOTE

- Atrial fibrillation
- Ventricular rate 153 bpm
- Some ST-segment depression in leads V_5–V_6: digoxin effect
- No other abnormalities

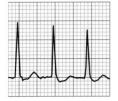

Rapid ventricular rate in lead V_6

THE ECG IN SYSTEMIC DISEASES

Cardiac involvement in a generalized disorder can cause arrhythmias and conduction defects, particularly if there is infiltration or the deposition of abnormal substances in the myocardium.

Thyroid disease

Thyrotoxicosis is probably the most common non-cardiac disorder that may present as a cardiac problem. It may cause atrial fibrillation, particularly in old age. There is usually a rapid ventricular response, which is difficult to control with digoxin (Fig. 8.10). An elderly patient may complain of palpitations or the symptoms of heart failure, and arterial embolization may occur. The usual symptoms of thyrotoxicosis may be mild or even absent.

Fig. 8.11

Fig. 8.12

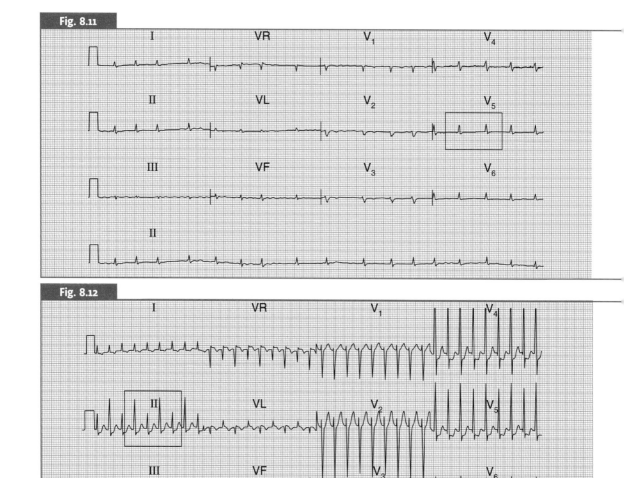

Malignant pericardial effusion
NOTE

- Atrial fibrillation
- Generally small QRS complexes
- Widespread T-wave flattening

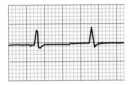

Small QRS complexes and flat T waves in lead V₅

Electrical alternans
NOTE

- Narrow complex tachycardia at 200 bpm (AVRNT)
- Alternate large and small QRS complexes

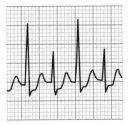

Alternate large and small QRS complexes in lead II

Malignancy

Metastatic deposits in and around the heart can cause virtually any arrhythmia or conduction disturbance. Malignancy is the most common cause of a large pericardial effusion, and a combination of atrial fibrillation and small complexes on the ECG suggest a malignant pericardial effusion. The ECG in Fig. 8.11 is from a 60-year-old man with metastatic bronchial carcinoma.

In the case of large pericardial effusions, with each beat the heart can rock within the effusion, causing alternate large and small QRS complexes. This is called 'electrical alternans'. The ECG in Fig. 8.12 is from another patient with carcinoma of the bronchus, who presented with a supraventricular tachycardia. Electrical alternans suggests the presence of a pericardial effusion, although in this case the QRS complexes are of normal size.

THE EFFECTS OF SERUM ELECTROLYTE ABNORMALITIES ON THE ECG

Although abnormal levels of serum potassium, magnesium and calcium can affect the ECG, the 'classical' changes are rarely seen. Occasionally, an ECG may suggest that the electrolytes should be checked, but the range of normality in the ECG is so great that an ECG is an unrealistic guide to electrolyte balance. Box 8.2 lists the possible causes of electrolyte imbalance, and Table 8.1 summarizes the ECG changes that may occur.

Potassium

Hyperkalaemia may cause arrhythmias, including ventricular fibrillation or asystole; flattening of the P waves; widening of the QRS complexes; depression or loss of the ST segment; and, particularly, symmetrical peaking of the T waves. The ECG in Fig. 8.13 is from a patient with renal failure and a potassium level of 7.4 mmol. After correction of the plasma potassium level, sinus rhythm was restored and the T waves were no longer peaked (Fig. 8.14).

BOX 8.2 Causes of Electrolyte Imbalance

Hyperkalaemia
- Renal failure
- Potassium-retaining diuretics (amiloride, spironolactone, triamterene)
- Angiotensin-converting enzyme inhibitors
- Liquorice
- Bartter's syndrome

Hypokalaemia
- Diuretic therapy
- Antidiuretic hormone secretion

Hypercalcaemia
- Hyperparathyroidism
- Renal failure

- Sarcoidosis
- Malignancy
- Myeloma
- Excess vitamin D
- Thiazide diuretics

Hypocalcaemia
- Hypoparathyroidism
- Severe diarrhoea
- Enteric fistulae
- Alkalosis
- Vitamin D deficiency

Fig. 8.13

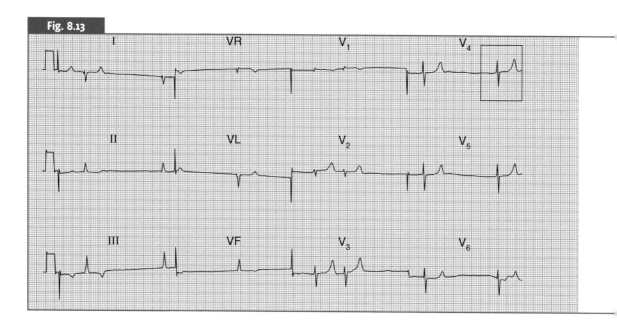

TABLE 8.1 The Effects of Electrolyte Imbalance on the ECG

Electrolyte	Effect of abnormal serum electrolyte level on ECG	
	Low level	High level
Potassium or magnesium	Flat T waves	Flat P waves
	Prominent U waves	Widening of QRS complexes (nonspecific intraventricular conduction delay)
	Depressed ST segment	Tall peaked T waves
	Prolonged QT interval	Disappearance of ST segment
	First or second degree block	Arrhythmias
Calcium	Prolonged QT interval (due to long ST segment)	Short QT interval, with loss of ST segment

Hyperkalaemia

NOTE

- No P waves
- Atrial fibrillation
- Junctional escape rhythm
- Right axis deviation
- Symmetrically peaked T waves, especially in the chest leads
- Inverted T waves in leads III, VF

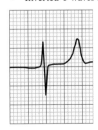

P wave absent and peaked T wave in lead V$_4$

Fig. 8.14

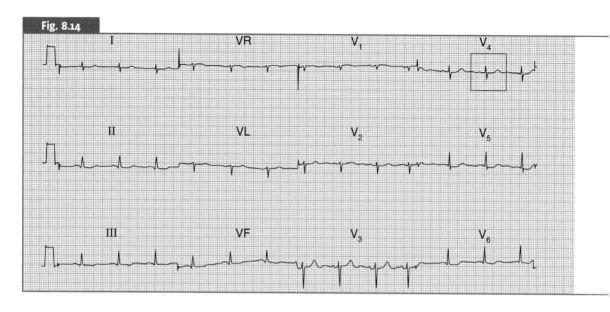

Fig. 8.15

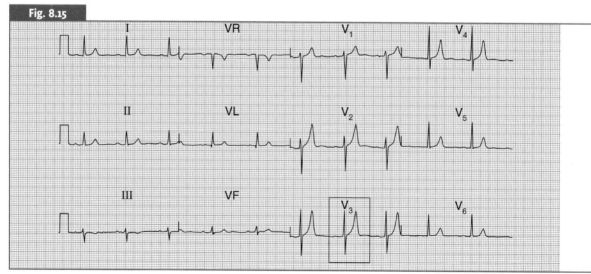

Remember, however, that peaked T waves are also a common finding in completely healthy patients (Fig. 8.15).

Hypokalaemia is common in patients with cardiac disease who are treated with powerful diuretics. It causes flattening of the T waves, prolongation of the QT interval, and the appearance of U waves. The ECG in Fig. 8.16 was recorded from a patient with severe heart failure due to ischaemic heart disease. The serum potassium level fell to 1.9 mmol, as a result of loop diuretic treatment without either potassium supplementation or the concomitant administration of an angiotensin-converting enzyme inhibitor.

Hyperkalaemia corrected

NOTE

- Same patient as in Fig. 8.13
- Sinus rhythm
- ST segment depression in inferior lateral leads
- Normal T wave configuration

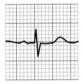

Normal P and T waves in lead V₄

Normal ECG

NOTE

- Sinus rhythm
- Normal axis
- Tall peaked T waves, resembling hyperkalaemia

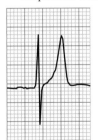

Tall, peaked T wave in lead V₃

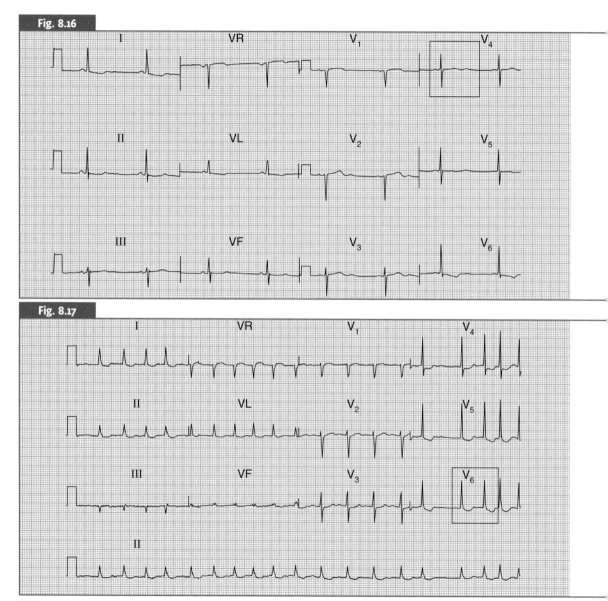

Fig. 8.16

Fig. 8.17

<hr>

Hypokalaemia

NOTE

- Leads V_1–V_6 recorded at half sensitivity
- Atrial fibrillation
- Normal axis
- Normal QRS complexes
- Flat T waves, with U waves in leads V_4–V_5

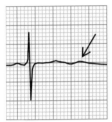

U wave in lead V_4

<hr>

Digoxin effect

NOTE

- Atrial fibrillation
- Normal axis
- Normal QRS complexes
- Downward-sloping ST segments in leads V_5–V_6

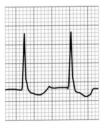

Downward-sloping ST segment in lead V_6

Magnesium

The effects of high and low serum magnesium levels on the ECG are essentially the same as those of high and low potassium levels.

Calcium

Hypercalcaemia shortens, and hypocalcaemia prolongs, the QT interval. However, the ECG remains normal within a very wide range of serum calcium levels.

THE EFFECTS OF MEDICATION ON THE ECG

Digoxin

Atrial fibrillation (AF) is normally associated with a rapid ventricular response (sometimes inappropriately called 'fast AF'), unless conduction through the atrioventricular node is slowed by medication. Digoxin, although no longer the firstline treatment, is still an effective drug for controlling the ventricular rate in atrial fibrillation. The dose can be critical: the first sign of toxicity may be a loss of appetite, and then the patient feels sick and vomits. Rarely, the patient complains of seeing yellow (xanthopsia). The main effect of digoxin on the ECG is downward sloping of the ST segments, especially in the lateral leads. The appearance is sometimes referred to as a 'reverse tick' (Fig. 8.17).

Fig. 8.18

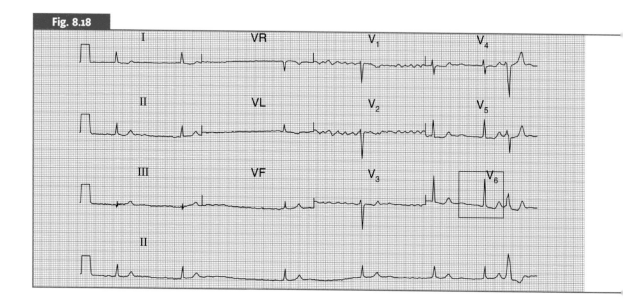

With increasing doses of digoxin the ventricular rate becomes regular and slow, and eventually complete heart block may develop. Digoxin can cause almost any arrhythmia, but especially ventricular extrasystoles and sometimes ventricular tachycardia. There is only a loose correlation between the symptoms and the ECG signs of digoxin toxicity.

The ECG in Fig. 8.18 was recorded from a patient with a congestive cardiomyopathy which caused atrial fibrillation and heart failure. She was vomiting and her failure had deteriorated, her heart rate having fallen to about 40 bpm.

The ECG in Fig. 8.19 shows another example of digoxin toxicity, which caused syncopal attacks due to runs of ventricular tachycardia.

The effects of digoxin on the ECG are listed in Box 8.3.

Drugs that prolong the QT interval

Many drugs have been reported to cause QT interval prolongation (Fig. 8.20) or torsade de pointes ventricular tachycardia (Fig. 8.21). See also Ch. 2, p. 72, and Ch. 4, p. 131. Drug withdrawal is usually required in affected patients.

Lithian

This can cause T wave changes such as those shown in Fig. 8.22 but this is not necessarily an indication to discontinue treatment if measured drug levels are acceptable.

Digoxin toxicity

NOTE

- Atrial fibrillation with one ventricular extrasystole
- Ventricular rate 41 bpm
- Normal QRS complexes
- Digoxin effect on ST segments in lead V$_6$

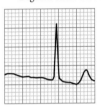

Downward-sloping ST segment in lead V$_6$

BOX 8.3 Effects of Digoxin on the ECG

- Downward sloping ST segments
- Flattened or inverted T waves
- Short QT interval
- Almost any abnormal cardiac rhythm, but especially:
  - sinus bradycardia
  - paroxysmal atrial tachycardia with AV block
  - ventricular extrasystoles
  - ventricular tachycardia
  - any degree of AV block
- Regularization of QRS complexes in atrial fibrillation suggests toxicity

---

Fig. 8.19

Digoxin toxicity

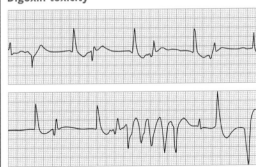

NOTE

- Continuous record
- Basic rhythm is atrial fibrillation: upright QRS complexes are probably the normally conducted beats
- Each upright QRS complex is followed by a predominantly downward complex, which represents a ventricular extrasystole
- Short run of ventricular tachycardia towards the end of the recording

Fig. 8.20

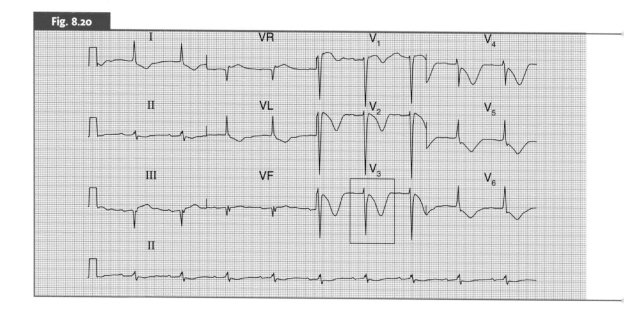

Fig. 8.21

Torsade de pointes VT

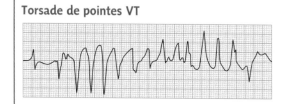

NOTE

- A single sinus beat is followed by a run of torsade de pointes ventricular tachycardia
- In this case the cause was a class Ia antiarrhythmic drug

Prolonged QT interval due to amiodarone

NOTE

- Sinus rhythm
- First degree block
- Normal QRS complexes
- QT interval 600 ms
- Widespread T-wave inversion

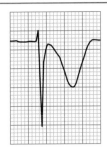

Long QT interval and inverted T wave in lead V_3

OTHER CAUSES OF AN ABNORMAL ECG

Trauma

Myocardial damage can be caused by chest injuries, either penetrating (e.g. stab wound) or closed (usually due to a steering wheel or seat belt). Direct trauma to the front of the heart can lead to occlusion of the left anterior descending coronary artery, and so to an ECG resembling that of an acute anterior myocardial infarction. However, seat belt injuries are more usually associated with myocardial contusion, as was the case in a young woman whose ECG is shown in Fig. 8.23.

Metabolic diseases

Most metabolic diseases, e.g. Addison's disease, are associated with nonspecific ST-segment or T-wave changes. There may be no apparent abnormality in the serum electrolytes. The ECG in Fig. 8.24 is from a young girl with severe anorexia nervosa: her serum electrolytes and thyroid function were perfectly normal – the ECG changes presumably reflect an intracellular electrolyte abnormality.

Cerebrovascular accidents

The association of a cerebrovascular accident and ECG abnormalities may suggest that the neurological problem

Fig. 8.22

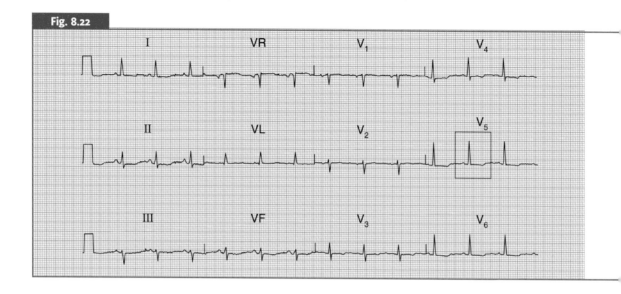

Fig. 8.23

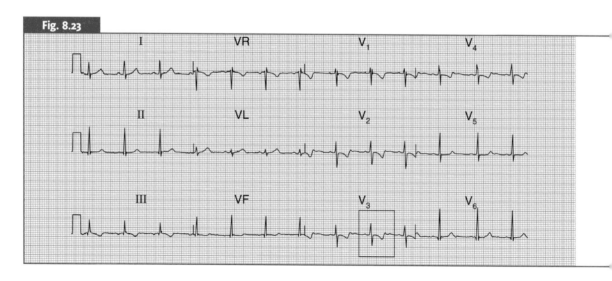

is secondary to a cerebral embolus, which can arise in the heart because of an arrhythmia, such as atrial fibrillation, or a left ventricular thrombus.

Sudden intracerebral events, particularly subarachnoid haemorrhage, can cause widespread T-wave inversion. The ECG in Fig. 8.25 is from a patient with subarachnoid haemorrhage.

Muscle disease

Many of the neuromuscular disorders are associated with a cardiomyopathy. The ECG in Fig. 8.26 is from a young man with no cardiovascular symptoms and a clinically normal heart, who had Friedreich's ataxia.

Lithium treatment
NOTE
- Sinus rhythm
- Normal axis
- Normal QRS complexes
- Normal QT interval
- Widespread T-wave inversion

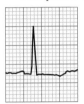

Inverted T wave in lead V₅

Trauma
NOTE
- Sinus rhythm
- Normal axis
- Partial RBBB pattern
- Anterior T-wave inversion

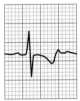

Inverted T wave in lead V₃

Fig. 8.24

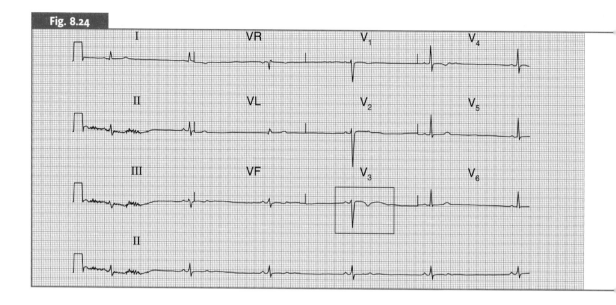

Fig. 8.25

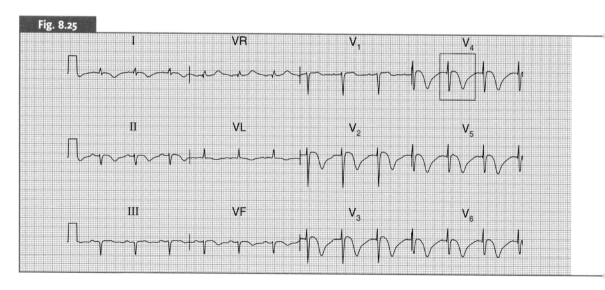

Anorexia nervosa
NOTE
- Sinus rhythm at 32 bpm
- Artefacts in leads II–III
- Normal axis
- Normal QRS complexes
- T-wave inversion and U waves in anterior chest leads

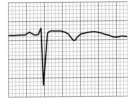

Inverted T wave and U wave in lead V₃

Subarachnoid haemorrhage
NOTE
- Sinus rhythm
- Left axis deviation
- QT interval 600 ms
- Widespread T-wave inversion

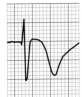

Long QT interval and inverted T wave in lead V₄

Fig. 8.26

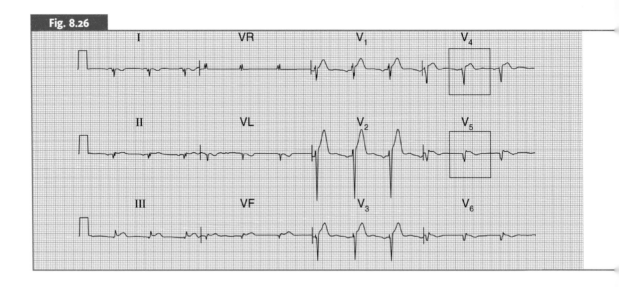

Friedreich's ataxia

NOTE

- Sinus rhythm
- Right axis deviation
- Widespread T-wave abnormality
- Appearances could suggest anterolateral ischaemia

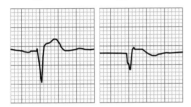

Changes in leads V_4 and V_5 suggesting an anterior infarction

Conclusions: four steps to making the most of the ECG

9

Description	313
Interpretation	314
Diagnosis	315
Treatment	315
Conclusion	316
Now test yourself	316

The theme of this book has been that the ECG is just one way of helping with the management of patients. The ECG is not an end in itself, and must always be seen in the context of the patient from whom it was recorded. To make the most of an ECG you need to think in four steps:
1. Describe it.
2. Interpret it.
3. See how it helps with the diagnosis.
4. Ask how it helps with treatment.

DESCRIPTION

An ECG can be described by anyone with the most basic knowledge, and an accurate description is needed as a basis for the later steps. The description starts with the heart rate and regularity, as measured by the intervals between the QRS complexes. The P waves must be identified; and if there are none, a clear statement of their absence is necessary. The relationship of the P waves to the QRS complexes is the next logical step, and the PR interval must be measured. The shape of the P wave needs to be recorded if it is abnormally peaked or bifid.

The QRS complexes need to be described in terms of their width and height, and also their shape: whether Q waves are present; whether there is more than one R wave in the QRS complex; and whether there are S waves in the leads where they would be expected. If there are Q waves, are they small and narrow, and are they only seen in the lateral leads, where they may be due to septal depolarization? If there are pathological Q waves, in which leads are they present, and do they suggest a possible inferior or anterior myocardial infarction? The cardiac axis should be defined.

Elevation or depression of the ST segment must be noted. If the ST segment is elevated, does it follow an S wave, so indicating high take-off? The T waves must be inspected in each lead, and while inversion in VR and V_1 is always normal, inversion in any other leads should be recorded. The QT interval should be measured, and if it appears long, it should be corrected for heart rate.

All these features can be identified without any knowledge of the patient, or indeed much knowledge of cardiology. The description of an ECG is reasonably well done by the automatic 'interpretation' function built into most modern ECG recorders, but it is important to remember that these are far from perfect. Automatic recorders tend to over-interpret ECGs so that nothing of importance is missed, and their descriptions are not always totally accurate. They can be poor at identifying P waves and they often miss ST-segment changes, and sometimes T-wave inversion. Therefore, you should never depend solely on a description provided by the ECG recorder itself.

INTERPRETATION

Always establish the cardiac rhythm first, because it may influence your interpretation of the rest of the ECG. For example, ventricular tachycardia, with its broad QRS complexes, will prevent any further interpretation – as will the broad complexes of complete heart block. The rhythm is established from the presence or absence of P waves and their relationship to the QRS complexes, from which arrhythmias and conduction defects can be accurately identified. On the whole, this part of ECG interpretation can be independent of the patient.

Otherwise, the accurate interpretation of an ECG should depend on knowledge of the patient. If the ECG has been recorded from a healthy subject, or a patient with no clinical suggestion of cardiac disease, then it is essential to remember the range of normality of the ECG. First degree block, and supraventricular or ventricular extrasystoles, are commonly seen in healthy people. P waves can be bifid in healthy people; right axis deviation can be normal in tall thin people; and minor degrees of apparent left axis deviation with a narrow QRS complex can occur in obese people and in pregnancy. An RSR[1] pattern with a normal QRS complex duration in lead V_1 is perfectly normal, and in some perfectly normal people there can be a small dominant R wave in lead V_1. Tall QRS complexes are frequently seen in healthy young people, and do not in themselves indicate left ventricular hypertrophy. Septal Q waves may be present in leads VL and V_5–V_6. Inverted T waves in the anterior chest leads can be normal in black people, while in white people they may be due to hypertrophic cardiomyopathy. Peaked T waves are often of no significance at all, although they can be due to hyperkalaemia.

In a patient with chest pain, however, the interpretation of the same ECG abnormalities can be quite different. T-wave inversion in the anterior chest leads may indicate a non-ST elevation myocardial infarction (NSTEMI). Left bundle branch block may be the result of an old or new infarction. A change of cardiac axis to the right may be due to a pulmonary embolism. A dominant R wave in lead V_1 might be due to a posterior myocardial infarction.

In a patient with breathlessness, right axis deviation, a dominant R wave in lead V_1 or T-wave inversion in leads V_1–V_3 may indicate multiple pulmonary emboli or idiopathic pulmonary hypertension. A deep S wave in lead V_6 may be due to chronic lung disease or to a pulmonary embolus. In patients complaining of attacks of dizziness, a finding such as first degree block, of little significance in a healthy subject, might indicate transient episodes of higher degrees of block causing a symptomatic bradycardia. A prolonged QT interval might point to episodes of torsade de pointes ventricular tachycardia.

Any described abnormality in an ECG must therefore be interpreted in the context of a knowledge of the patient's condition; otherwise, ECG changes will support a less focused differential diagnosis.

DIAGNOSIS

The ECG is essential for the diagnosis of problems involving rhythm and conduction, in which the interpretation and the diagnosis are clearly strongly linked. However, it is necessary to remember that the identification of a specific arrhythmia does not complete the diagnosis, which should include the cause of the arrhythmia. For example, the cause of atrial fibrillation may be ischaemic or valvular heart disease, or alcoholism, or thyrotoxicosis, or a cardiomyopathy, and so on. Heart block may be due to idiopathic His bundle fibrosis, but it also raises the possibility of ischaemic or hypertensive heart disease. Left bundle branch block may be due to aortic stenosis, and right bundle branch block may be associated with an atrial septal defect.

ECG appearances that suggest faults in the recording technique may sometimes point to a clinical diagnosis. For example, artefacts due to movement may suggest a neurological disorder such as Parkinson's disease. Low-voltage QRS complexes may be due not to poor standardization but to obesity, emphysema, myxoedema or a pericardial effusion.

An ECG cannot diagnose the presence of heart failure, although with a totally normal ECG, heart failure is unlikely. The ECG may, however, help in diagnosing the cause of heart failure, which is often the key to treatment – atrial fibrillation, ventricular hypertrophy or left bundle branch block may suggest valve disease, or there may be evidence of an old myocardial infarction. Similarly, the ECG is not a good way of identifying electrolyte abnormalities, but flat T waves, U waves, and long QT intervals should at least suggest the possibility that there may be an electrolyte problem. A long QT interval, on the other hand, may be due to one of the congenital syndromes or to one of a wide variety of drugs.

The accurate identification of an ECG abnormality is thus only part of the diagnostic process: we still need to determine the underlying cause. The ECG often points the way to appropriate further investigations, such as chest X-rays, echocardiography, blood tests for electrolyte abnormalities, or cardiac catheterization, and the ECG is simply part of the diagnostic process.

TREATMENT

The ECG is obviously paramount in determining the treatment of an arrhythmia or conduction defects. It is also crucial for the proper use of acute interventions in both ST elevation myocardial infarction (STEMI) and NSTEMI. But its limitations must also be understood; in particular, it must be remembered that the ECG can be normal in the early stages of a myocardial infarction, and a normal, or near-normal, ECG is not an adequate reason for sending a patient with chest pain home from an accident and emergency (A&E) department.

Without an understanding of the ECG, devices such as pacemakers and implanted cardioverter defibrillators (ICDs) could not have been invented. These devices, and the techniques that use them, such as dual chamber pacing and cardiac resynchronization therapy (CRT), are the province of the specialist. But as the devices and techniques become increasingly prevalent, they will be encountered more and more often by general practitioners and specialists in non-cardiac disciplines. For example, patients with these devices tend to be elderly, and it is the elderly who most frequently experience multiple medical problems – so non-cardiac specialists are bound to come across patients who have problems, but who also have a modern electrical device that is working perfectly normally.

CONCLUSION

The ECG is easy to describe and interpret, but it is often more difficult to appreciate the range of normality, and to remember that a full diagnosis encompasses the cause of any abnormality that may have been identified. The ECG is an essential part of the overall diagnostic process in a wide variety of patients, and in some it influences treatment. The most important thing to remember is that diagnosis and management depend on a full consideration of the individual patient, not just of the ECG.

Now test yourself

150 ECG Cases, a companion to this volume, gives 150 clinical scenarios with full related ECGs, and poses questions about ECG interpretation and the diagnosis and management of patients.

Index

Page numbers followed by "*f*" indicate figures, "*t*" indicate tables, and "*b*" indicate boxes.

A

'A' wave, 161–163, 164*f*
AAI. *see* Right atrial pacemakers
Abnormal ECG
  abnormal muscle movement and, 283, 284*f*
  artifacts in, 283–285
  cerebrovascular accidents and, 305–307, 308*f*
  congenital heart disease and, 285–291, 285*b*
  effects of medication on, 301–302
  hypothermia and, 283–285, 284*f*, 286*f*–287*f*
  metabolic disease and, 305, 308*f*
  muscle disease and, 307, 310*f*
  serum electrolyte abnormalities and,
    295–301
  subarachnoid haemorrhage and, 307, 308*f*
  in systemic diseases, 293–295
  trauma and, 305, 306*f*
Accelerated idionodal rhythm, 48*f*, 95, 95*f*
  Lown-Ganong-Levine syndrome *vs*, 69–72
Accelerated idioventricular rhythm, 29*f*, 95, 95*f*
Accessory pathway, 69, 100
  ablation of left-sided, 137*f*
Acute coronary syndromes, 198–199
Acute myocardial infarction, temporary pacing
  in patients with, 163
Addison's disease, 305
AH interval, 161–163
Ambulatory ECG recording (Holter), 62, 85–87
  monitoring devices, 89*f*, 89*t*
Amiodarone
  prolonged QT interval due to, 74*f*, 305*f*
  torsade de pointes ventricular tachycardia
    and, 302, 304*f*
Aneurysm, left ventricular, 209
Angina. *see also* Chest pain
  ECG in, 198
  Prinzmetal's 'variant', 229
  stable, 198–199
  unstable, 198–199
Anorexia nervosa, 305, 308*f*

Antiarrhythmic drugs
  prolonged QT interval due to, 304*f*
  torsade de pointes ventricular tachycardia
    and, 304*f*
Anti-tachycardia pacing, 143
Anxiety
  breathlessness and, 255
  sinus tachycardia of, 257
Aortic dissection, 197*b*
Aortic regurgitation, 198, 256*b*
Aortic stenosis, 235, 256*b*, 288*f*, 289
  left bundle branch block with, 263, 263*f*
  severe, left ventricular hypertrophy with,
    264, 264*f*
  syncope, 62, 63*f*–64*f*
Arrhythmia, 57–58
  amenable to ablation, 138–141
  arterial pulse in, 94*t*
  breathlessness and, 257
  digoxin and, 302
  electrophysiology, 93
  exercise testing discontinuation, 246
  heart rates associated, 93, 94*t*
  management, 133
  syncope due to, 59*b*
Artefacts, in ECG, 315
  recordings, 283–285
Arterial pulse, in arrhythmias, 94*t*
Asystole, 58–59, 61*f*
Athletes, ECG in, 48*f*, 49, 49*b*, 50*f*–52*f*
Atrial extrasystoles, 7, 99, 213*f*
Atrial fibrillation, 111, 112*f*, 156*f*
  ablation, 138, 140*f*
  anterior ischaemia with, 226*f*, 227
  causes of, 111*b*
  complete heart block with, 156*f*, 158*f*
  with coupled ventricular extrasystoles, 258
  digoxin effect on, 300*f*, 301–302, 302*f*–303*f*
    ischaemia and, 241–244, 243*f*
  in hyperkalaemia, 296*f*
  in hypokalaemia, 300*f*

inferior infarction and, 126*f*
with left bundle branch block (LBBB), 116*f*,
  117
in malignancy, 294*f*, 295
management
  digoxin control of ventricular rate of, 302
  intermittent VVI pacing, 177*f*
  pacing, 164
in mitral stenosis, 68, 256*b*
paroxysmal, 68, 86*f*
in pulmonary embolism, 231, 233
with right bundle branch block (RBBB),
  122*f*
with slow ventricular rate, 148*b*, 154,
  155*f*–156*f*
syncope, 148*b*
in thyroid disease, 292*f*, 293
in thyrotoxicosis, 292*f*
uncontrolled, 258
Atrial flutter, 107–109, 108*f*
  with 1 : 1 conduction, 109, 110*f*
  with 2 : 1 block, 108*f*
  with 4 : 1 block, 109, 110*f*
  ablation, 138, 139*f*
  hypothermia and, 284*f*, 285, 286*f*–287*f*
  intermittent VVI pacing, 174*f*
  slow ventricular rate, 154, 155*f*–156*f*
  with variable block, 155*f*
Atrial pacing, 185, 187
  spike, 182*f*
Atrial septal defect, 290*f*
  right bundle branch block with, 291, 293*f*
Atrial tachycardia, 105, 106*f*
  re-entry and enhanced automaticity, 98*f*
Atrial tracking, 186*f*
Atrioventricular block, 157–163, 160*f*
  endocardial ECGs, 161–163
Atrioventricular nodal escape, 154*f*
Atrioventricular nodal re-entry tachycardia
  (AVNRT), 104*f*, 105, 106*f*
  re-entry and enhanced automaticity, 98*f*

Atrioventricular re-entry tachycardia, 100–103, 101*f*
Atrium
  automatic depolarization frequencies, 77–78
  silent, 151, 152*f*
Automatic recorders, in ECG, 314
Automaticity, 77–78
  enhanced, 95
    re-entry and, differentiation between, 97, 98*f*
  rhythms resulting from, 77–78
AV node ablation, 138–141
AVNRT. *see* Atrioventricular nodal re-entry tachycardia

B

Bicycle ergometer, 245
Bifascicular block, 83*f*
Bigeminy, 99
Biventricular hypertrophy, congenital heart disease and, 285*b*
Biventricular pacemaker, 193*t*
Biventricular pacing, 280, 280*f*
Black people, ECG of
  inverted T waves in, 314
  normal, T wave inversion, 235
Blood flow obstruction, syncope due to, 59*b*
Blood pressure, exercise testing and, 246
Bradycardia, 2
  ECG, 147–191, 148*f*
  management of, 163–191
    dual chamber pacemakers (DDD), 184*f*, 185–188, 193*t*
    permanent pacing, 163–170
    right atrial pacemakers (AAI), 182*f*, 183, 193*t*
    right ventricular pacemakers (VVI), 170–179, 171*f*, 193*t*
    temporary pacing, in patients with acute myocardial infarction, 163
  mechanism of, 147–163, 148*b*
    atrial fibrillation/flutter, 154, 155*f*–156*f*
    AV block, 157–163, 160*f*
    sinoatrial disease, 147–153, 150*f*, 152*f*
  palpitations/syncope symptoms, 77–79
    ECG between attacks, 77
  syncope due to, 59*b*, 147
Bradycardia-tachycardia syndrome, 153*f*
  sick sinus syndrome, 153*f*
Breathlessness, 255–281
  atrial fibrillation

    with coupled ventricular extrasystoles, 258, 258*f*
    uncontrolled, 258
  atrial septal defect and, 291
  biventricular pacing in, 280, 280*f*
  cardiac resynchronization therapy in, 278–281, 279*b*, 279*f*–280*f*
  causes of, 255, 256*b*
  chronic lung disease in, 276, 276*f*
  chronic obstructive pulmonary disease in, 273*b*
  disorders affecting the left side of the heart, 259–267
    left atrial hypertrophy, 259, 260*f*–261*f*
    left ventricular hypertrophy, 259–267, 263*f*–264*f*, 266*f*, 268*f*, 271*f*
  disorders affecting the right side of the heart, 269–278, 271*b*, 273*b*
    right atrial hypertrophy, 269–272, 270*f*, 272*f*
    right ventricular hypertrophy, 272–278, 272*f*, 274*f*, 275*t*, 276*f*
  history and examination of, 255–257
  hypertrophic cardiomyopathy, 268, 268*f*
  ischaemia, 266, 266*f*
    left ventricular hypertrophy, 266, 266*f*
  left anterior hemiblock, 268, 268*f*
  left bundle branch block, with aortic stenosis, 263, 263*f*
  mitral stenosis, 260, 260*f*
  normal variant, 274, 274*f*
  pulmonary embolism in, 271*b*, 276, 276*f*
  pulmonary hypertension, 260, 260*f*
  rhythm problems in, 257, 258*f*
  Wolff-Parkinson-White syndrome, 271, 271*f*
Broad complex tachycardia, 73*f*
  associated with Wolff-Parkinson-White syndrome, 133, 134*f*
  capture beats, 127–130, 128*f*
  differentiation of, 130, 131*b*
  fusion beats, 127–130, 128*f*
  irregular, 117
    atrial fibrillation in, 111, 112*f*
  in myocardial infarction, 113–115
  P waves, 114*f*, 115–117, 116*f*
  QRS complex, 119–127, 119*f*–122*f*, 125*f*–126*f*, 129*f*
  supraventricular, 113, 114*f*
  of uncertain origin, 125*f*
  ventricular, 119*f*–121*f*
    supraventricular, 125*f*

Broad QRS complex
  pacing spike followed by, 172*f*
  with RV apical pacing, 181*f*
Bruce protocol, 245, 245*t*
Brugada syndrome, 76*f*, 77
Bundle of Kent, 68–69, 100

C

CAD. *see* Coronary artery disease
Calcium, imbalance in, 295, 297*t*, 301
Capture beats, broad complex tachycardia, 127–130, 128*f*
Cardiac arrest, 141–144
Cardiac axis, 14*f*, 15–17
  in ECG, 314
  'leftward limit' of normality, 19*f*
  right axis deviation, 16*f*
  'rightward' limit of normality, 16*f*
Cardiac memo, 89*f*, 89*t*
Cardiac resynchronization therapy (CRT), 193*t*, 278–281, 279*f*, 315
  ECG appearance in, 278–281, 280*f*
  indications for, 278, 279*b*
  specialist functions of, 281
Cardiac rhythm, 314
  abnormalities of, due to re-entry, 96, 97*f*
  normal, 2, 2*f*–3*f*
  in sick sinus syndrome, 149*b*
Cardiomyopathy, congestive, 302
Carotid sinus hypersensitivity, 59*b*
Catheter ablation, 95, 135–138
  arrhythmias amenable to, 138–141
  atrial fibrillation, 138, 140*f*
  atrial flutter, 138, 139*f*
  AV node, 138–141
  left-sided accessory pathways, 136–138, 137*f*
  mapping/ablation catheter (MAP), 136–138, 137*f*
  paroxysmal atrial fibrillation, 138
  pathway, 141
  ventricular tachycardia, 141
Cerebrovascular accidents, abnormal ECG and, 305–307, 308*f*
Chest pain, ECG in, 195–253, 314
  acute, 195–198
    causes of, 196*b*
    features of, 195, 197*b*
    presence of, 198
  angina, 244
  causes of, 195, 196*b*, 235

chronic, 244
    causes of, 196*b*
    investigation of, 245–253
    ECG pitfalls in, 235–253
        false negatives/positives, 235–237
        R wave changes, 236*f*, 237–241, 239*f*
        ST segment and T wave changes,
            239*f*–240*f*, 241–244, 242*f*–244*f*
        ST elevation, 235–237
        summary, 237*b*
    exercise testing *see* Exercise testing
    history and examination of, 195–198
    left ventricular hypertrophy, 235
    management of, 253
    pericarditis, 235
    pulmonary embolism, 195, 196*b*
    recurrent, causes of, 196*b*
    ST segment depression and, 225, 227
    of unknown cause, 198–199
Chest X-rays
    fractured pacing lead, 189*f*
    of pacemaker assessment, 163
    right atrial/ventricular lead displacement, 188*f*
Children, ECG in, 52, 53*b*
Chronic lung disease, 276, 276*f*
Chronic obstructive pulmonary disease, 273*b*
Clockwise rotation, 19–21
Complete (third degree) block, 79, 83*f*
    atrial fibrillation with, 154, 158*f*
    AV block, 157, 158*f*
    Stokes-Adams attack, 157–161, 160*f*
    VVI pacing, 177*f*
Complete heart block, 177*f*
    with atrial fibrillation, 156*f*, 158*f*
Conduction
    anterograde (normal), 68–69
    delay, 101*f*
    normal, 68, 100, 101*f*
    re-entry, 68, 100, 101*f*
    retrograde, 78, 100
Conduction defects, 77
Congenital heart disease, ECG in, 285–291
    appearance of, 285*b*
Congenital long QT syndrome, 73, 74*f*–75*f*
Congestive cardiac failure, 257
Cor pulmonale, 257
Coronary artery disease (CAD), prevalence of,
    247, 247*b*
Coronary spasm, 229
Coupled ventricular extrasystoles, atrial
    fibrillation with, 258
Creatine kinase, CK-MB, 198
CRT. *see* Cardiac resynchronization therapy

D

DDD. *see* Dual chamber pacemakers
Defibrillation, CRT device, 193*t*
Delta wave, 68–69
Delta wave, in Wolff-Parkinson-White
    syndrome, 271*f*
    type A, 69, 70*f*, 72*b*, 237–241, 239*f*
    type B, 72*f*, 239*f*, 241
Depolarization, 68, 77–78
    atrial, 77–78
    endocardial ECG, 161–163
    late, 95
    normal, 68, 77–78
    pacemaker action, 164–165
    reversed, 96
    spontaneous (automaticity), 77–78
    Wolff-Parkinson-White syndrome, 68–69
Dextrocardia, 12*f*
    leads reversed, 13*f*
Digoxin, 241–244, 243*f*
    arrhythmias and, 302
    atrial fibrillation and, 302, 302*f*
    ECG diagnostic pitfalls, 236*t*
    effects of, on ECG, 300*f*, 301–302,
        303*b*
    enhanced automaticity and, 95
    ischaemia and, 241–244, 243*f*
    ST segment depression, 241–244, 243*f*
        downward-sloping, 236*t*, 241–244,
            243*f*
    ST segments in, downward-sloping, 300*f*,
        301, 302*f*–303*f*
    T wave inversion, 241–244, 243*f*
    toxicity of, 302, 302*f*–303*f*
Dizziness, 58–59
    ECG in, 314
    exercise testing discontinuation, 246
    sick sinus syndrome, 147–149
Drugs, prolonged QT interval, 73, 74*f*
    amiodarone, 74*f*
Dual chamber pacemakers (DDD), 184*f*,
    185–188, 193*t*
    atrial pacing with ventricular tracking,
        187
    atrial tracking, 186*f*
    ECG appearance, 185–187, 186*f*
    indications for, 185*b*
    magnet rate, 191, 192*f*
    pacing: intermittent, 187*f*
    rate response (DDDR), 188
    specialist functions of, 188
Dual chamber pacing, 315

E

Ebstein's anomaly, 290*f*, 291
    right atrial hypertrophy and right bundle
        branch block in, 290*f*
ECG
    in athletes, 48*f*, 49, 49*b*, 50*f*–52*f*
    in children, 52, 53*b*
    four steps of, 313–316
        conclusion in, 316
        description in, 313–314
        diagnosis in, 315
        interpretation in, 314–315
        treatment in, 315
    in healthy people, 1–55
        types of, 1–2, 2*f*–4*f*
    normal, 53–54
Ectopic atrial rhythm, 7, 8*f*
Elderly, thyroid disease in, 292*f*, 293
Electrical alternans, 294*f*, 295
Electrical pulse, 164
Electrogram, normal His bundle, 162*f*
Electrolyte abnormalities
    ECG in, 315
    effects on ECG of, 295–301
Electrophysiology, 93
    catheter ablation, 135–138
    complications of, 142*b*
    endocardial ECG, 135, 136*f*
    indications of, 141, 142*b*
    mapping/ablation catheter (MAP), 136–138,
        137*f*
    purpose of studies, 93
    scale of traces, 136–138
    tachycardia, 135–141
    transvenous catheters during, 136*f*
Emphysema, QRS complexes in, 315
Endocardial ECG, 135, 136*f*
    in AV block, 161–163
Enhanced automaticity, 95
    catheter ablation, 135–136
    re-entry and, differentiation between, 97,
        98*f*
Escape beats, 61*f*, 78
    junction, 6*f*
    junctional, 78
    ventricular, 79*f*
Escape rhythms, 77–78, 147
'Event recorders', 85
Exercise
    ischaemia induced by, 247, 248*f*
    normal ECG, pre-, 252*f*, 253
    ST segment elevation induced by, 247, 251*f*

319

Exercise *(Continued)*
   ventricular extrasystoles induced by, 252*f*, 253
   ventricular fibrillation induced by, 253, 253*f*
Exercise-induced tachycardia, 130*f*, 131
Exercise testing
   Bruce protocol for, 245, 245*t*
   contraindications of, 251*b*
   discontinuation reasons on, 246–247
   'false positive', 246–247
   interpretation of ECG during, 247
   ischaemia, 247, 248*f*
   normal, 247, 247*b*, 248*f*
   'positive', 247
   practical aspects of, 245–246
   risk of, 247–253
   sensitivity/specificity, 247
   ST segment depression, 247, 251*f*
   ventricular extrasystole development, 252*f*, 253
   ventricular fibrillation development, 253, 253*f*
Extrasystoles, 5–7, 57, 95
   atrial, 7, 99, 213*f*
   causing symptoms, 98*f*, 99, 100*f*–101*f*
   enhanced automaticity causing, 95
   healthy people, 87
   junctional, 5, 99
   supraventricular, 5, 8*f*
   ventricular, 7, 10*f*

F

Fallot's tetralogy, 291
   right ventricular hypertrophy in, 291*f*
'False positive,' exercise testing, 246–247
Fascicular tachycardia, 122, 122*f*
First degree block, 79, 152*f*, 160*f*, 163*f*
   His electrogram, 163*f*
   left bundle branch block, 79, 80*f*
   RBBB and left anterior hemiblock with, 83*f*
   RBBB with, 152*f*
Flutter waves, in lead II, 155*f*
Friedreich's ataxia, 307, 310*f*
Fusion beats, broad complex tachycardia, 127–130, 128*f*

G

Garment worn ECG monitor, 90*t*–91*t*

H

'H' spike, 161–163
Haemorrhage, subarachnoid, 307, 308*f*
Heart block, 314–315
   causes of, 162*b*
   complete, 158*f*
   trifascicular block, 83*f*
Heart failure, 257
Heart rate, 2–5
   arrhythmia, 93, 94*t*
   control, 77–78
   exercise testing and, 246
     discontinuation indication, 246
   maximum, calculation, 246
   sinus or paroxysmal tachycardia, 57–58
Herpes zoster, 197*b*
His bundle
   orthodromic tachycardia, 103
   re-entry circuit involving, 68
   re-entry tachycardia and, 100
   in trifascicular block, 79, 83*f*
His bundle electrogram
   normal, 162*f*
   of second degree block, 163, 164*f*
     2:1 block, 163
His bundle fibrosis, 315
His bundle systems, slow conduction through, 154
His pacemakers, 179, 179*f*–181*f*
His pacing system, 179*f*–180*f*
Holter monitor, 89*f*, 89*t*
HV interval, 161–163
Hypercalcaemia, 296*b*, 301
Hyperkalaemia, 295, 296*b*, 296*f*, 298*f*
   corrected, 298*f*
Hypertrophic cardiomyopathy, 66*f*, 268, 268*f*
   ECG diagnostic pitfalls, 236*t*
   ECG features, 66*f*
   ECG with, 267
   MR image, 66*f*
   syncope due to, 59*b*, 66*f*
Hypocalcaemia, 296*b*, 301
Hypokalaemia, 296*b*, 299, 300*f*
Hypothermia, 283–285, 284*f*, 287*f*
   atrial flutter in, 284*f*, 285, 286*f*–287*f*
   rewarming after, 286*f*

I

ICD. *see* Implanted cardioverter defibrillator
Idioventricular rhythm, accelerated, 95, 95*f*

Implantable loop recorder, 89*f*, 89*t*
Implanted cardioverter defibrillator (ICD), 141–144, 315
   abnormal function, 143–144
   anti-tachycardia pacing, 143
   chest X-ray, 141
   defibrillator function, 141–143
   dual chamber (DDD/ICD), 193*t*
   ECG appearance, 143
   indications for, 143
     insertion, 143*b*
   pacemaker function, 141
   single chamber, 141, 144*f*
   subcutaneous, 141, 145*f*
   ventricular fibrillation, 141–143, 145*f*
Infants, normal ECG in, 285
Infection, 197*b*
Inspiration, normal ECG during, 40*f*
Intracardiac recordings, 161
Intrinsic beat
   atrial sensing and ventricular pacing, 187*f*
   first and second, 177*f*
Ischaemia, 225–227, 266, 266*f*
   anterior, 224*f*, 225
     atrial fibrillation with, 226*f*, 227
     AV nodal re-entry tachycardia with, 227, 229*f*
       inferior infarction and RBBB with, 219, 222*f*
       RBBB with, 219, 221*f*
   anterolateral, 225, 227*f*
     Friedreich's ataxia and, 310*f*
   diagnosis by exercise testing, 247, 248*f*
   digoxin effect *vs.*, 241–244, 243*f*
   lateral, 202*f*
   left ventricular hypertrophy *vs.*, 240*f*, 241, 266, 266*f*
   myocardial, ECG in, 198–229
   normal variant confusion, 235
   without myocardial infarction, 225–227
Isolated tricuspid stenosis, 269–271, 270*f*

J

J point, 199–200
J wave, 283, 284*f*, 286*f*–287*f*
Jugular venous pulse, in arrhythmias, 94*t*
Junctional escape beat, 6*f*, 78, 78*f*
Junctional escape rhythm, 78, 78*f*–79*f*
   hyperkalaemia and, 296*f*
   sustained, 78
Junctional (AV nodal) extrasystoles, 5, 99

Junctional region, automatic depolarization frequencies, 77–78
Junctional tachycardia, with bundle branch block, 114*f*
  right, 122*f*

L

Large ventricular pacing spike, 174*f*
LBBB. *see* Left bundle branch block
Leadless, pacemakers, 178, 178*f*
Left anterior hemiblock, 79, 83*f*, 268, 268*f*
  RBBB and, 79, 80*f*, 83*f*
Left atrial hypertrophy, 11, 68*f*
  ECG in, 259, 260*f*–261*f*
  left ventricular hypertrophy and, 261, 261*f*
  mitral stenosis, 68
Left axis deviation
  acute anterolateral infarction with, 208*f*, 209, 210*f*
  anterior NSTEMI, 222*f*, 223
  bifascicular block, 83*f*
  congenital heart disease and, 285*b*
  trifascicular block, 83*f*
Left bundle branch block (LBBB), 56*t*, 64*f*, 219
  with aortic stenosis, 263, 263*f*
  atrial fibrillation with, 116*f*, 117
  causes of, 219*b*
  myocardial infarction with, 218*f*, 219
Left coronary artery, normal/occluded, 205*f*, 207*f*
Left main stem coronary artery, 205*f*, 207*f*
  narrowing of, 241
Left ventricular aneurysm, 209
Left ventricular hypertrophy, 234*f*, 235, 240*f*, 241, 263–264, 263*f*–264*f*
  aortic dissection and, 235
  aortic stenosis, syncope due to, 62, 63*f*–64*f*
  congenital heart disease and, 285, 285*b*, 288*f*, 289
  ECG in, 259–265, 263*f*–264*f*
    mimic, 265–267, 266*f*, 268*f*, 271*f*
  ECG pitfalls, 236*t*
  ischaemia, 266, 266*f*
  lateral ischaemia *vs.*, 241
  left atrial hypertrophy and, 261, 261*f*
  with severe aortic stenosis, 264, 264*f*
Lithium treatment, ECG and, 306*f*
Long QT syndrome, 72–73
  congenital, 73, 74*f*–75*f*
  drug toxicity, 133*f*
  genetic abnormalities, 73, 74*f*–75*f*
  syncope due to, 59*t*
Loop recorder, 89*f*, 89*t*
Lown-Ganong-Levine syndrome, 69–72, 72*f*
Lung disease, 197*b*

M

Magnesium, abnormal levels of, 297*t*, 301
Magnet rate, pacemakers, 191, 192*f*
MAP. *see* Mapping/ablation catheter
Mapping/ablation catheter
Mapping/ablation catheter (MAP), 136–138, 137*f*
Marked right ventricular hypertrophy, 272, 272*f*
Medication
  effects of, on the ECG, 301–302
  prolonged QT interval and, 302, 305*f*–306*f*
Metabolic disease, abnormal ECG and, 305, 308*f*
Metabolic equivalents (METs), workloads expressed in, 246, 246*b*
METs. *see* Metabolic equivalents
Mini loop recorder, 90*t*–91*t*, 91*f*
Mitral regurgitation, 256*b*
Mitral stenosis, 68, 68*f*, 256*b*
  atrial fibrillation, 68
  left atrial hypertrophy, 68
  pulmonary hypertension and, 260, 260*f*
Mitral valve prolapse, 256*b*
Mobile phone apps, 90*f*, 90*t*–91*t*
Muscle movement, abnormal, 283, 284*f*
Myocardial infarction, 197*b*
  acute, 199*b*
  anterior, 203–211, 205*f*
    acute, and old inferior infarction, 215, 216*f*
    NSTEMI, 222*f*, 223
    old, 209–211, 210*f*
    old, acute inferior infarction with, 214*f*, 215
    old inferior infarction with, 215, 216*f*
    poor R wave progression, 214*f*
    RBBB with, 219, 221*f*
    V2-V5 leads, 203, 205*f*
  anterolateral, 209
    acute, 208*f*, 209
    acute, with left axis deviation, 208*f*, 209
    age unknown, 209, 210*f*
    old, 209–211, 210*f*
    old, NSTEMI, 241, 242*f*
  CABG-related, 199*b*
  criteria for, 199*b*
  definition of, 198
  diagnosis/ECG, 198, 237*b*
  ECG changes, sequence of features, in STEMI, 199–219
  ECG pitfalls in, 236*t*, 237*b*
  false positives/negatives, 237*b*
  inferior, 200–203
    acute, 201*f*, 214*f*
    anterior ischaemia with, 214*f*, 215
    anterior NSTEMI with, 217*f*
    evolving, 202*f*–203*f*
    old, acute anterior infarction with, 215, 216*f*
    old, anterior ischaemia with, 224*f*, 225
    RBBB and possible anterior ischaemia with, 219, 222*f*
    right ventricular infarction, 213
  lateral, 203–211
    acute, 207*f*
    after 3 days, 203, 208*f*–209*f*
    LBBB with, 218*f*, 219
    multiple, 214*f*, 215, 216*f*–217*f*
    PCI-related, 199*b*
    posterior, 211, 213*f*
      dominant R wave in lead V₁, 211, 213*f*
      old, 236*f*, 237
    prior, criteria for, 199*b*
    secondary to ischaemia, 198
    serial ECG recordings, 211
    ST segment elevation, causes of, 34*b*
    subendocardial, 223
    types of, 199*b*
    without ischaemia, 225–227
Myocardial perfusion scintigraphy, 245
Myxoedema, QRS complexes in, 315

N

Narrow complex tachycardias, causing symptoms, 99–111, 99*b*
Nonspecific ST segment/T wave changes, 197*f*
Non-ST elevation myocardial infarction (NSTEMI), 67, 198–199, 222*f*, 223, 241, 314
  acute inferior infarction with, 215, 217*f*
  anterior, 198–199, 222*f*, 223
  ECG changes in, 223–229
  hypertrophic cardiomyopathy *vs*, 67
  old anterolateral, 241, 242*f*
  STEMI *vs.*, 223

Normal ECG, 2–54, 2f
  in adults, 54b
  in black people, 235
  cardiac axis, 14f, 15–17
  endocardial, 161–163
  exercise testing, 247, 250f
  extrasystoles, 5–7, 8f, 87
  heart rate, 2–5
  P wave, 9–11
    inverted, 9, 12f
    notched or bifid, 11, 14f
    peaked, 11
  PR interval, 13
  Q wave, 235
  QRS complex, 14f, 15–31, 16f
  QT interval, 75f
  R wave, dominant wave in lead V₁, 236f, 237
  right ventricular hypertrophy and, 236t
  supraventricular extrasystoles, 5
  T wave inversion, in black people, 235
  variants, ischaemia vs., 235, 236t
  ventricular extrasystole, 7, 10f
Normal PR interval, 182f
Normal QRS complex, 182f
Normal variant, 274, 274f
NSTEMI. see Non-ST elevation myocardial
    infarction

O

Obesity, QRS complexes in, 314–315
Oesophageal rupture, pain, 197b
Orthodromic tachycardia, 102f–103f, 103
Orthopnoea, 257
Oxygen, rate of use, metabolic equivalents, 246

P

P wave, 9–11, 10f, 160f
  absent, in hyperkalaemia, 295, 296f
  bifid, 63f
    in left atrial hypertrophy and left
        ventricular hypertrophy, 261f
    in mitral stenosis and pulmonary
        hypertension, 260f
  broad complex tachycardia, 114f, 115–117,
      116f
  complete heart block of, 160f
  dextrocardia, 9, 12f–13f
  following QRS complex, junctional escape
      rhythm, 78, 78f

inverted, 9, 10f, 12f
  junctional escape rhythms, 78, 78f–79f
    in lead V₁, 158f
    in lead VL, 158f
  left atrial hypertrophy, 68f
  nodal rhythm overtaking, accelerated
      idionodal rhythm, 95, 95f
  normal ECG, 10f
  notched or bifid, 11, 14f
  pacing spike following, 186f
  peaked, 11
    Ebstein's anomaly, right atrial hypertrophy
        and right bundle branch block
        and, 290f
    pulmonary embolism, 231, 232f
    right atrial hypertrophy, 11
    in right atrial hypertrophy, 270f, 272f
    in right ventricular hypertrophy, 272f
Pacemakers, 163
  abnormal function, 188–191
  failed pacing capture, 188–189, 190f
  failure, 188
  functions of, 141, 163–164
  indications for, 191
  interrogation, 165f
  leadless, 178, 178f
  magnet rate, 191, 192f
  monitoring, 165, 165f–166f, 168f
  nomenclature, 165–170
  over-sensing or far-field sensing, 189, 191f
  single-chamber, 164–165
  tachycardia mediated, 189, 192f
  types of, 170t, 193t
  under-sensing, 189, 190f–191f
Pacing
  bipolar, 164, 172f
  description of, 164
  failed capture, 188–189, 190f
  intermittent, DDD, 187, 187f
  permanent, 163–170
  temporary, in acute myocardial infarction,
      163
  unipolar, 164
  VVI bipolar, 172f
Pacing lead, 164, 179, 189f
  atrial, 184f
  displacement, 188f
Palpitations, 57–79
  ambulatory ECG, 85–87, 89t
  bradycardia causing, 77–79
    ECG between attacks, 77
    escape rhythms, 77–78
  clinical history and diagnosis, 57–62, 59b, 59t

diagnosis of cause, 62
  ECG features, between attacks, 62–79, 63t
  paroxysmal tachycardia, 58t
  physical examination, 62
  sinus tachycardia, 58t
  tachycardias causing, 58t, 68–77
    Brugada syndrome, 76f, 77
    long QT syndrome, 72–73
    mitral stenosis, 68, 68f
    pre-excitation and Wolff-Parkinson-White
        syndromes, 68–72
  thyroid disease and, 293
Parkinsonism, 283, 284f
Paroxysmal tachycardia, diagnosis from
    symptoms, 58t
Paroxysmal ventricular tachycardia, 72
Partial RBB pattern, trauma and, 306f
Partial right bundle branch block, 26f, 27
Patch ECG monitor, 90f, 90t–91t
PCI. see Percutaneous coronary interventions
Peaked T waves, 314
Percutaneous coronary interventions (PCI),
    myocardial infarction related to, 199b
Pericardial effusion
  malignant, 294f, 295
  QRS complexes in, 315
Pericardial pain, 197b
Pericarditis, 196b, 198, 234f, 235
Pneumothorax, 197b
Post-cardioversion, 126f
Postural hypotension, 59b
Post-ventricular atrial refractory period
    (PVARP), 189
Potassium, abnormalities in, 295–299, 296f,
    297t, 300f
PR interval, 13
  in ECG, 313
  prolonged
    first degree block, 80f
    trifascicular block, 83f
  short
    Lown-Ganong-Levine syndrome, 69–72,
        72f
    in Wolff-Parkinson-White syndrome,
        271f
    Wolff-Parkinson-White syndrome type
        A, 70f, 72b
    Wolff-Parkinson-White syndrome type
        B, 70f, 72f
Pre-excitation syndromes, 68–72
Pregnancy, ECG in, 52, 52b, 314
Prinzmetal's variant angina, 228f, 229
Prolonged QT interval, in lead V₄, 157f

Pulmonary embolism, 196b, 271b, 276, 276f
  ECG abnormalities in, 231
  ECG in, 198, 230f–233f, 231
  pain, 196b–197b
  right axis deviation, 231, 231f–232f
  T wave inversion, 231, 231f–232f
Pulmonary hypertension, 260, 260f
  thromboembolic, 65, 231
Pulmonary stenosis, 288f
PVARP. see Post-ventricular atrial refractory
  period

Q

Q wave, 31
  in ECG, 313–314
  inferior infarction and RBBB and anterior
    ischaemia, 219, 222f
  myocardial infarction, 199, 199b
    acute anterior and old inferior infarctions,
      214f, 215
    acute inferior and old anterior, 215, 216f
    acute inferior STEMI, 201f
    acute inferior STEMI and anterior
      (NSTEMI), 215, 217f
    acute lateral STEMI, 207f
    evolving inferior STEMI, 202f
    inferior and right ventricular infarction,
      213
    lateral STEMI (3 days old), 208f–209f
    posterior infarction, 211, 213f
  normal, 30f, 33f
  in normal ECG, 33f
  septal, 235
QRS complex, 26f, 27
  alternate large and small, 294f, 295
  broad, in left bundle branch block with
    aortic stenosis, 263f
  broad complex tachycardia, 119–127,
    119f–122f, 125f–126f, 129f
  in ECG, 313–314
  narrow paced, 180f
  normal ECG, 29f–30f
  normal variant, 27, 29f
  slurred upstroke (delta wave), 70f
  small, in malignancy, 294f
  tall, 242f
  Wolff-Parkinson-White syndrome, 68–69,
    70f
QT interval, 47, 48f
  correction for heart rate (QT$_c$), 73
  in ECG, 314

normal, posterior infarct with, 74f
prolonged, 72, 75f
  amiodarone causing, 74f
  causes, 73, 74f, 75b
  drugs causing, 302, 305f–306f
  hypocalcaemia and, 301
  subarachnoid haemorrhage and, 308f
  unexplained, with T wave abnormality,
    240f, 241
QT$_c$
  long QT syndrome, 73
  sudden death risk and, 73

R

R on T phenomenon, 99, 101f
  in healthy people, 87
R wave
  chest leads, 19–21, 20f, 22f–24f, 26f
  dominant, 21, 24f
    in probable normal variant, 274f
  dominant in lead V$_1$, 237–241, 239f
    normal ECG, 236f, 237
    old posterior infarction, 236f, 237
    posterior infarction, 211, 213f
    pulmonary embolism, 231
    right ventricular hypertrophy, 237
    Wolff-Parkinson-White type, 237–241,
      239f
  Ebstein's anomaly, right atrial hypertrophy
    and right bundle branch block and,
    290f
  ECG interpretation pitfalls and, 236f, 237
  in hypertrophic cardiomyopathy, 268f
  in marked right ventricular hypertrophy,
    272f
  normal ECG, 24f, 26f
  poor progression, anterior infarction,
    209–211, 210f, 214f, 215
  pulmonary stenosis and, 288f
  right ventricular hypertrophy, 64f, 275t
  slurred upstroke (delta wave), 237–241, 239f
  tall, left ventricular hypertrophy, 63f, 234f,
    263f–264f
RBBB. see Right bundle branch block
Re-entry, cardiac rhythm abnormalities due
  to, 96, 97f
  tachycardia, 68
Re-entry pathway, 68
  enhanced automaticity and, differentiation
    between, 97, 98f
  in pre-excitation syndromes, 96, 97f

Repolarization, 241
  delayed, 72
Reverse tick, 301
Right atrial hypertrophy, 270, 270f, 272, 272f
  congenital heart disease and, 285b
  in Ebstein's anomaly, 290f, 291
  in Fallot's tetralogy, 291f
  in peaked P waves, 11
Right atrial pacemakers (AAI), 182f, 183, 193t
  chest X-ray, 188f
  ECG appearance, 182f, 183
  indications for, 183b
  pacing, 182f
  rate response modulation (AAIR), 183
Right axis deviation
  in chronic lung disease, 276
  in ECG, 314
  Friedreich's ataxia, 310f
  in hyperkalaemia, 296f
  in marked right ventricular hypertrophy, 272
  in mitral stenosis and pulmonary
    hypertension, 260
  pulmonary embolism, 231, 231f–232f
  pulmonary stenosis and, 288f
  in right atrial and right ventricular
    hypertrophy, 272
  in right ventricular hypertrophy, 274f, 275t
Right bundle branch block (RBBB), 56t, 219
  acute inferior infarction with, 218f, 219
  anterior myocardial infarction with, 219,
    221f
  atrial fibrillation with, 122f
  with atrial septal defect, 291, 293f
  Brugada syndrome, 77
  congenital heart disease and, 285b, 290f,
    291, 293f
  in Ebstein's anomaly, 290f, 291
  with first degree block, 152f
  first degree block with, 83f
  inferior myocardial infarction with possible
    anterior ischaemia, 219, 222f
  left anterior hemiblock and, 83f
  long PR interval and, 152f
  in lead V$_1$, 160f
  partial, trauma and, 306f
  pattern, partial, 260
Right coronary artery, normal vs. occluded,
  201f
Right ventricular hypertrophy, 64f, 272–278,
  272f, 274f, 275t, 276f
  chest pain and, 236t
  congenital heart disease and, 285, 285b, 288f,
    289, 290f, 291

Right ventricular hypertrophy *(Continued)*
　ECG pattern of, 231
　marked, 272, 272*f*
　normal variant *vs.*, 236*t*
　pattern in pulmonary hypertension, 231
　thromboembolic pulmonary hypertension,
　　65
Right ventricular infarction, 212*f*–213*f*, 213
　acute, 213
　inferior infarction with, 213
Right ventricular outflow tract ventricular
　　tachycardia (RVOT-VT), 95, 96*f*
Right ventricular pacemakers (VVI), 170–179,
　　171*f*, 193*t*
　bipolar pacing, 172*f*
　ECG appearance, 172–173, 172*f*, 174*f*, 177*f*
　functions of, 178
　indications for, 173*b*, 193*t*
　intermittent pacing, 177*f*
　　atrial flutter with, 177*f*
　rate response modulation (VVIR), 178
　unipolar, 174*f*
R-R interval, sinus rhythm, 2
RSR pattern
　pulmonary embolism, 231, 233*f*
　RBBB and acute inferior infarction, 218*f*,
　　219
　RBBB and anterior infarction, 219, 221*f*
RSR¹ pattern
　Brugada syndrome, 76*f*
　in ECG, 314
RV apical pacing, 180*f*–181*f*
RVOT-VT. *see* Right ventricular outflow tract
　　ventricular tachycardia

S

S wave
　acute anterolateral infarction with left axis
　　deviation, 208*f*
　chest leads, 19–21, 20*f*, 22*f*–24*f*
　deep
　　in atrial fibrillation with coupled
　　　ventricular extrasystoles, 258*f*
　　in left bundle branch block with aortic
　　　stenosis, 263*f*
　in ECG, 313–314
　normal ECG, 24*f*
　persistent
　　in chronic lung disease, 276*f*
　　in pulmonary embolism, 231, 231*f*, 276*f*
　　in pulmonary stenosis, 288*f*

　in right atrial hypertrophy, 272*f*
　in right ventricular hypertrophy, 272*f*
R wave size balance, 17, 18*f*–19*f*, 19–21
Second degree block, 148*b*, 158*f*, 162*b*, 163,
　　164*f*
　of 2 : 1, 164*f*
　　His bundle electrogram, 162*f*, 163
　of 3 : 1, 157, 158*f*
　　His bundle electrogram, 163
Seizures, 58–59, 59*t*
Sensing, by pacemakers, 164–165
Septal Q waves, 314
Shingles, pain, 197*b*
'Sick sinus' disease, 148*b*
Sick sinus syndrome, 147–153, 150*f*, 152*f*
　acquired, 155*b*
　bradycardia-tachycardia syndrome, 153*f*
　cardiac rhythms in, 149*b*
　causes of, 155*b*
　familial, 155*b*
　pacing, VVI, 173*b*
　sinus bradycardia, 148*f*
'Silent atrium', 151, 152*f*
Single chamber implanted cardioverter
　　defibrillator (ICD) devices, 141, 144*f*
Single-chamber pacemaker, 164–165
Sinoatrial disease, 147–153, 150*f*, 152*f*
Sinoatrial node, 77–78
　abnormal function of, 147–149
Sinus arrest, 151, 151*f*, 154*f*
Sinus arrhythmia, healthy people, 2
Sinus bradycardia, 5, 6*f*, 7*b*, 56*t*, 147, 148*f*, 150*f*
Sinus pauses, 87*f*, 149, 150*f*
Sinus rhythm, 2, 3*f*, 5*b*, 7*b*
　following cardioversion, 106*f*, 108*f*
　with left bundle branch block (LBBB), 114*f*,
　　115
　with normal conduction, 126*f*
　syncope causes associated, 58–59
　Wolff-Parkinson-White syndrome, type A,
　　103*f*
Sinus tachycardia, 93
　diagnosis from symptoms, 58*t*
　in healthy people, 2–5, 6*f*, 56*t*
　palpitations due to, 57
　pulmonary embolism, 231*f*–232*f*
Sodium channels, abnormal, Brugada
　　syndrome, 77
Spasm, of coronary arteries, 229
Spinal pain, 197*b*
ST segment, 35, 36*f*
　chest pain diagnosis, pitfalls, 239*f*–240*f*,
　　241–244, 242*f*–244*f*

depression
　anterior ischaemia, 224*f*, 225, 226*f*–227*f*,
　　227, 229*f*
　digoxin causing, 241–244, 243*f*
　exercise test discontinuation, 246
　exercise testing, 247, 248*f*
　horizontal, in ischaemia, 225, 247
　posterior infarction, 211, 213*f*
　unstable angina, 198–199
downward-sloping
　digoxin and, 241–244, 243*f*, 300*f*, 301,
　　302*f*–303*f*
　raised, Brugada syndrome, 76*f*
in ECG, 314
ECG interpretation pitfalls, 239*f*–240*f*,
　　241–244, 242*f*–244*f*
elevation of, 203
　multiple infarctions, 215, 217*f*
　myocardial infarction (STEMI), 198–219
　pericarditis, 234*f*, 235
　persistent, 209
high take-off, 235, 240*f*
in lead V₃, 34*f*
in lead V₄, 33*f*–34*f*
in left ventricular hypertrophy with severe
　　aortic stenosis, 264*f*
nonspecific changes in myocardial
　　infarction, 197*f*
normal ECG, 36*f*, 38*f*–39*f*, 247, 250*f*
raised
　acute anterior and old inferior infarction,
　　214*f*, 215
　acute inferior infarction, 200–203, 201*f*,
　　214*f*
　acute lateral infarction, 203, 207*f*
　anterior infarction, 205*f*
　inferior and right ventricular infarction,
　　213
　multiple infarctions, 214*f*, 215,
　　216*f*
　posterior infarction, 211, 213*f*
upward-sloping, 251*f*
STEMI, 198–219
　acute inferior, 200–203, 201*f*
　　anterior NSTEMI with, 215, 217*f*
　acute lateral, 203, 207*f*
　anterior, 203–211
　definition/criteria of, 198–199
　lateral, 203–211, 208*f*–209*f*
　NSTEMI *vs.*, 223
　old anterior infarction, 209–211, 210*f*
　sequence of features characteristic of,
　　199–200

Stokes-Adams attack, 59b, 157–161, 160f
Stress MRI, 245
Subarachnoid haemorrhage, 236t, 307, 308f
Subcutaneous implanted cardioverter defibrillator (ICD) devices, 141, 145f
Subendocardial infarction, 223
Sudden death, 59t
  long QT syndrome and, 72–73, 74f–75f
Supraventricular extrasystoles, 5, 8f, 98f, 99
Supraventricular tachycardia, 102f
  ambulatory ECG, 87
  broad complex tachycardia, 113, 114f
Syncope, 57–59
  cardiovascular causes, 59b, 62–67
    aortic stenosis, 62, 63f–64f, 63t
    arrhythmias, 59b, 62
    hypertrophic cardiomyopathy, 66f, 67
    mitral stenosis, 68, 68f
    pre-excitation syndromes causing, 68–72
    pulmonary emboli, 65
  definition/meaning, 58
  diagnosis of causes, 59, 59t
  ECG features between attacks, 62–79, 63t, 85–87
  long QT syndrome causing, 72–73
  neurally-mediated syndromes, 59b
  physical examination, 62
  tachycardia, 68–77
    ECG between attacks, 68–77
Systemic diseases, ECG in, 293–295
Systolic pressure, exercise testing discontinuation, 246

T

T wave, 38f–40f, 39–47, 231
  chest pain diagnosis, pitfalls, 239f–240f, 241–244, 242f–244f
  in ECG, 314
  flat, in hypokalaemia, 299, 300f
  flattened, 44f, 46f
  flattening, nonspecific, 197f, 244, 244f
  inversion, 40f, 41b, 43f–44f, 241
    acute inferior (STEMI) and anterior (NSTEMI) infarction, 215, 217f
    anterior, 235, 241
    anterior NSTEMI, 222f, 223
    digoxin effect, 241–244, 243f
    hypertrophic cardiomyopathy, 66f, 67
    inferior infarction, 201f–202f

ischaemia, 241
  lateral, 241, 242f
  lateral infarction, 209f
  in lead III, 197f
  left bundle branch block, 64f
  left ventricular hypertrophy, 63f, 234f, 236f, 240f, 241
  long QT interval and, 240f, 241
  nonspecific changes in myocardial infarction, 197f
  NSTEMI, 199, 223, 231f
  pulmonary embolism, 231, 231f–232f
  right ventricular hypertrophy, 64f
  unexplained T wave abnormality with, 240f, 241
  Wolff-Parkinson-White syndrome, type A, 70f
  Wolff-Parkinson-White syndrome, type B, 70f, 72f, 239f
inverted
  amiodarone and, 305f
  in hypertrophic cardiomyopathy, 268f
  in left anterior hemiblock, 268f
  in left ventricular hypertrophy, 263f–264f
  in probable ischaemia, 266f
  pulmonary stenosis, 288f
  in right ventricular hypertrophy, 274f, 275t
  trauma and, 306f
in left ventricular hypertrophy, with severe aortic stenosis, 264f
maximal, in left ventricular hypertrophy, ischaemia, 266f
peaked, 46f, 47
  in healthy patients, 298f, 299
  hyperkalaemia and, 295, 296f
in prolonged QT syndrome due to amiodarone, 74f
unexplained abnormality, 240f, 241
Tachycardia, 2, 93–144
  antidromic reciprocating, 103
  carotid sinus pressure, 105
  exercise-induced, 130f, 131
  fascicular, 122, 122f
  management of, 133
  mechanism of, 93–133
    enhanced automaticity and triggered activity, 95, 95f–96f
    re-entry, abnormalities or cardiac rhythm due to, 96, 97f
    re-entry mechanisms, 68

non-paroxysmal, 95
  orthodromic, 102f–103f, 103
  pacemaker-mediated, 189, 192f
  palpitations and syncope symptoms, 68–77
  paroxysmal, 58t
  reciprocating, 103
  re-entry and enhanced automaticity, differentiation between, 97, 98f
  right ventricular outflow tract ventricular, 130f, 131
  symptoms
    broad complex tachycardia causing, 113–130, 113b, 114f
    extrasystoles causing, 98f, 99, 100f–101f
    narrow complex tachycardias causing, 99–111, 99b
  syncope due to, 59b
  in Wolff-Parkinson-White syndrome, 69
'Tachycardia-bradycardia syndrome', 151
Third degree block, 148b
Thromboembolic pulmonary hypertension, 65, 231
Thyroid disease, 292f, 293
Thyrotoxicosis, 292f, 293
Torsade de pointes, ventricular tachycardia, 72–73, 73f, 131, 132f–133f
Transition point, 19
  shift in, pulmonary embolism, 231
Trauma, abnormal ECG and, 305, 306f
Treadmill, for exercise testing, 245
Trifascicular block, 83f
Trigeminy, 99
Triggered activity, 95, 96f
  catheter ablation, 135–136
Troponin, elevation, 198–199
  causes (not myocardial infarction), 198
  in myocardial infarction, 198, 199b
T wave abnormalities, 56t

U

U wave, 46f, 48f, 51f
  anorexia nervosa and, 308f
  in hypokalaemia, 299, 300f
Uncontrolled atrial fibrillation, 258
Unpaced beat, first and second, 174f

V

Valve disease, ECG in, 256b
Vasovagal attack, 7b, 59b, 147
Ventricular aneurysm, 209
Ventricular escape beat, 79f
Ventricular extrasystole, 7, 10f, 56t, 87, 99,
  100f–101f
  exercise-induced, 252f, 253
Ventricular fibrillation (VF), 141, 142f
  exercise-induced, 253, 253f
  implanted cardioverter defibrillator (ICD)
    devices, 141–143, 145f
Ventricular pacing, 172, 184f
  atrial, 184f

Ventricular tachycardia, 114f, 118f,
  130f
  ablation, 141
  ambulatory ECG recording, 87
  broad complexes, 119f–121f
  causes of, 115b
  digoxin toxicity and, 302f–303f
  episodes, in long QT syndrome,
    73
  fusion and capture beats, 128f
  inferior infarction and, 129f
  intermittent, 92f
  paroxysmal, 72
  prolonged QT syndrome with, 72
VVI. see Right ventricular pacemakers

W

Wandering pacemaker, 95
Wolff-Parkinson-White (WPW) syndrome,
  68–72, 237–241, 267, 271, 271f
  with atrial fibrillation, 133, 134f
  ECG diagnostic pitfalls, 236t
  ECG features summary, 69–72
  re-entry circuit, 100
  sinus rhythm, 70f, 72f
  type A, 69, 70f, 103f, 133, 134f, 237–241,
    239f
  type B, 69, 70f, 72f, 239f, 241
WPW syndrome see Wolff-Parkinson-White
  (WPW) syndrome